JASON VALE
THE JUICE MASTER

Juice
Yourself Slim

By the same author

Keeping it Simple – Over 100 Delicious Juices and Smoothies

7lbs in 7 Days Super Juice Diet

Turbo-charge Your Life in 14 Days

Chocolate Buster: The Easy Way to Kick Your Addiction

The Juice Master's Ultimate Fast Food: Discover the Power of Raw Juice

The Juice Master's Slim 4 Life: Freedom from the Food Trap

JASON VALE
THE JUICE MASTER

Juice
Yourself Slim

Lose Weight without Dieting

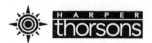

HARPER
thorsons

NB While the author of this book has made every effort to ensure that the information contained in this book is as accurate and up-to-date as possible at the time of publication, medical and pharmaceutical knowledge is constantly changing and the application of it to particular circumstances depends on many factors. This book should not be used as an alternative to specialist medical advice and it is recommended that readers always consult a qualified medical professional for individual advice before following any new diet or health programme. The author and publishers cannot be held responsible for any errors and omissions that may be found in the text, or any actions that may be taken by a reader, as a result of any reliance on the information contained in the text, which are taken entirely at the reader's own risk.

HarperThorsons
An Imprint of HarperCollins*Publishers*
77–85 Fulham Palace Road
Hammersmith, London W6 8JB

The website address is: www.thorsonselement.com

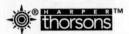

and *HarperThorsons* are trademarks
of HarperCollins*Publishers* Limited

Published by HarperThorsons 2008

10 9

© Jason Vale 2008

Jason Vale asserts the moral right to be
identified as the author of this work

A catalogue record for this book is
available from the British Library

ISBN-13 978-0-00-726714-9
ISBN-10 0-00-726714-2

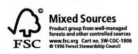

Mixed Sources
Product group from well-managed
forests and other controlled sources
www.fsc.org Cert no. SW-COC-1806
© 1996 Forest Stewardship Council
FSC

Contents

Introduction: Igniting the Fire Within   1

1   Juice Yourself *Super* Slim!   9
2   The Juice Revolution   30
3   The Appliance of Juicy Science   50
4   Environ Mental!   76
5   The Finest Health Insurance in the World   96
6   Exercising Your God-given Right to
    Better Health Insurance   106
7   *Changing Rooms* versus *Grand Designs*   114
8   The Simple Way   120
9   The Launch   131
10 Juice Yourself Slim *for Life*   136
11 The Launch Pack   150
12 Juice Yourself Slim *on the Move*   160
13 Super Boost Me!   165
14 Super-slimming Juices   171
15 Super-slimming Smoothies   200
16 Souper Slimming Fuel   231
17 Super-slimming Salads   252

Questions 'n' Answers   273
Recommended Juice and Smoothie Bars   285
Want to be a Juice Master Natural Juice Therapist?   287
Index   289

... a BIG thank you ...

I would like to thank all the people who made this book possible, from the publishers, the editor and the proof-reader to the lawyer! However, I reserve the biggest thank you to my mother and closest friend (who are one and the same person), all my other friends and of course Katie, who has been a rock of support throughout the writing of this book – thank you for everything.

Introduction

Igniting the Fire Within

When I wrote *Slim 4 Life: Freedom from the Food Trap* back in 2001, I honestly thought I would never need to write another book on slimming. At the time the book was groundbreaking. It was the first to distinguish clearly between 'normal' foods and what I coined 'drug' or 'junkie' foods. The book went on to become a bestseller and was talked about on television and radio. I soon started to receive thank-you letters and emails from just about every corner of the globe. The people who wrote to me not only had lost incredible amounts of weight in an extremely healthy way, but had also done so *effortlessly* – a breakthrough concept for most people who had tried to lose weight in the past.

Clearing the Brainwashing

Slim 4 Life slowly chipped away at the tremendous amount of brainwashing about food we have been subjected to since birth. By the time people had finished the book they simply couldn't see junk(ie) food or the industry in the same light again, no matter how hard they tried. This meant people went from a 'diet mentality' of 'I want but I *can't* have' – a mental state that creates feelings of deprivation, mood swings and ultimate failure – to the unique non-diet mentality of 'I *can* but I don't actually want.' This wonderful frame of mind eliminates any need for willpower. We need willpower only if we still crave food and drink we believe we can no longer have. However, if we genuinely have no desire for these 'foods' any more, there can be no internal mental battle.

This frame of mind is a slimmer's dream. It's the mindset where you see other people eating things like chocolate, chips or crisps, and instead of looking on in envy, you actually feel elated by the fact that you genuinely have no craving whatsoever for these foods and are pleased to be free of the slavery to them. It's the frame of mind where you even feel excited about eating healthily and exercising.

You may not have read *Slim 4 Life*, but I can almost guarantee that at some point in your life you have reached that wonderful slimming utopia mindset of feeling inspired and on fire. You may have been to a seminar, read a different book or just got there yourself.

Dousing the Flames

What I didn't realize when I first wrote *Slim 4 Life*, however, was that no matter how much you light someone's fire and inspire them to change there are many elements of life that can easily douse those flames. Before we know it we are back to square one – or to a *'round one'* if you will!

Whether it's work, relationships, hormones, the influence of others or the gradual drip-feed brainwashing by the drug food and drink industry, the inspirational fire we felt could never leave us suddenly loses its strength and, for some, appears to go out completely. I say *appears* because the beauty of being human is that no matter how much life may knock us off course, the pilot light is always on. It may be extremely dim, and to some may feel about as dead as it gets, but it's there, in all of us – and it's often relatively simple to reignite it.

For some people, this light never appears to dim. I know thousands of people who read *Slim 4 Life* and experienced a complete, unwavering life change. Equally, I know many people who read the book and felt completely elated and on fire and lost tremendous amounts of weight effortlessly – only to pile it all back on, and sometimes more! This leads to a feeling of utter frustration and cries of 'Why didn't I just keep with it?', 'What happened to that frame of mind?' and, most commonly, 'Why can't I get back to how I was thinking then?'

The Sixth Sense Syndrome

Many people try to relight the inspirational fire using the same method that helped them succeed before, such as rereading the book. I know people who have tried to reread *Slim 4 Life* or *Turbo Charge Your Life in 14 Days* in order to get exactly the same revelation they had the first time. However, they find that 'it just wasn't the same'. This is because you can't possibly have the same revelation twice. It's like the film *The Sixth Sense* with Bruce Willis. The first time you see it the twist at the end is a complete revelation, and the very aspect that makes the film what it is. However, those who watch it a second time can't possibly get the same revelation, and most tend to analyse the whole film, rather than going with the flow and enjoying it. The same principle applies to all 'self-help' books, and indeed a book like *Slim 4 Life*. The first time is a revelation for most, but the second reading is often a case of the person flicking through, hunting for the 'trigger' that will enlighten them again, analysing the book instead of reading it with the same intensity.

Sometimes it's worth rereading a book as you may well have missed things first time around, but this is *only* beneficial if you are already in the right frame of mind and just need a little reminder or retune. If, however, you achieve success but then lose the plot, the chances of the book being as effective are super slim. I know many people who read the infamous *Easy Way to Stop Smoking* by Allen Carr and found it easy to stop for a length of time but started smoking again. Many tried to reread the book only to find it wasn't anywhere near as effective as the first time. They needed a different way of receiving the same or similar information (like a session at one of his clinics) for them to see the light again and gain true freedom from smoking.

The Easy Way to the Land of the Slim

I now realize that, with food and diet, a mental boost to reignite the fire within at least once every year is essential for lifelong success. That is why I have written this book. One book or seminar is rarely enough, especially when it comes to permanent weight loss and supreme health. The amount of advertising, brainwashing, conditioning and peer pressure attached to the wrong kinds of foods and drinks cannot be ignored. It's this gradual dripping tap that eventually starts to dampen the fire, and before you know it you are heading down the road to fat land once again. Also, unlike with smoking or alcohol, we have associations with 'junkie' foods and drinks that go back to when we were just a year or two old. This means we have millions of associations with certain 'foods'. Tidy the room and we can have an ice cream. We hurt ourselves and are comforted with a cake, and so on. Even after months or years of change, these associations can easily return.

My aim for this book is twofold:

- ✿ To ignite or reignite the juicy fire within and put you in that glorious, inspired 'non-diet' frame of mind.
- ✿ To provide a new and *extremely easy* juice and lifestyle programme that is perfectly healthy and extraordinarily effective.

Juice Yourself Slim is the result of years of nutritional, psychological, diet and addiction research. It may appear simplistic, but that's part of its beauty. All the hard work has been done for you. The *only* thing you are required to do for slimming and health success is to read the whole book and follow the simple instructions. I have already set out the first instruction and, other than putting the programme into practice, it's the most important one. The instruction may sound obvious, but you will be amazed at how many people feel they will have as much success without carrying it out. That instruction is to actually read the book, in its entirety and in the order it was written.

The ONLY thing you need to do for slimming and health success is to read the whole of this book and follow the simple instructions.

The number of people who buy books of this nature but never read them – let alone act on them – is quite frightening. Every book I have ever written has this fundamental instruction at the start. I cannot emphasize enough just how important it is to read every word and not to flick through the book or jump directly to the programme, however tempting it is.

Often you will see that I repeat certain points. Many may not like the way I write or the 'basic English' I use to get my message across. This book is designed so that *anyone* can read it and anyone can get the results. I am not here to win any literary awards and I never, ever think of myself as an author. I write books, but I am not an author in the true sense of the word. This isn't about winning the Booker Prize; it's about results. And if we are all honest, even if you don't like the way I write but you get a flat stomach at the end of it – who cares!

Lay the Right Foundations

We live in an 'instant gratification' society. The days of effort equalling rewards appear to be numbered. Our natural tendency these days is to start to try building a new slim life without laying down any good foundations. However, without the right foundations things inevitably collapse, as you may have discovered in the past. Reading every page of this book is the equivalent to laying down good solid foundations. I have studied addiction, nutrition and hypnosis for years, and this book is a combination of information, motivation and a form of hypnosis. It has been designed to *gradually* penetrate both your conscious and subconscious mind. It has been written in this way to slowly remove a great deal of brainwashing about food, health, disease, the legal drug industry and nutrition in order to ignite that inner fire once again.

For those who are fearful of any kind of hypnosis, I wish to explain that most people are *already* living in hypnosis, and the idea of this book is simply to remove it in order to see things as they actually are. Those in the advertising industry know all about the power of unconscious hypnosis. You may feel that you choose the soap powder you use, the trainers you buy, the clothes you wear and indeed the food and drinks you consume. However, all too often these choices have been made for you. This is why it is essential to use similar techniques in order to remove the unconscious hypnosis so prevalent in the junkie food industry.

Not Juiced about Juicing Yourself Slim?

Part of the foundation process is to make sure you have more than one reason for introducing freshly extracted juices into your life. This is extremely important for life change. My mission is for juicing to become a daily part of your life, even *after* you get slim. If your only reason for juicing and smoothie-making is to get slim, the chances are that when you have reached your slim goal, you will have much less reason to juice on a regular basis. While slimming is clearly an extremely important part of this book (for some it's everything!), the effectiveness of fresh juices in treating and preventing disease plays a bigger role. This is why although this book is aimed at people wishing to slim in an extremely healthy way, it is also aimed at *already* slim people who need a mental and physical boost on the health front.

This book is for people wishing to slim healthily, but also for already slim people who need a mental and physical boost on the health front. My mission is for juicing to become a daily part of your life, even AFTER you get slim.

I have included many juice studies and stories within this book. Some of them are not directly related to being overweight. You may feel these aren't relevant to you as you 'just want to get on with it'. You may also think I repeat myself a lot. However, I cannot emphasize enough that everything in this book is there for a reason, even if at the time you may not see it. The repetition, as annoying as it can be, is essential to fully embed the message. I know that when you read the fascinating stories about the effectiveness of freshly extracted juices and smoothies, your brain will have many more reasons to get some of this wonderfully powerful liquid fuel into your system on a regular basis, regardless of whether you are slim or overweight.

For best results, make a point of reading a few pages just before you sleep and then on waking. I would certainly advise that you read some of the book on a daily basis. Once you put it down for a few days, it might be the end of it! So, even if the book starts to jar for whatever reason, do yourself a favour and keep on reading. There will be times when you will be itching to start. Some of the life-changing stories alone will make you want to start … NOW! However (and yes, I know I am labouring this point), wait until you are fully armed with all of the information.

If you follow this first instruction, which will give you the mental impetus to act on the information, you will be one of thousands who will go from eating themselves fat to juicing themselves slim!

One Last Thing …

In case you are worried you will have to spend hours in the kitchen chopping fruit and veg into a million pieces and cleaning the machine, let me put your mind at rest before we even start. Juicing has hit broadband status and you can now put three whole apples into the machine without peeling or chopping, and juicers now go in the dishwasher! The plan I have devised is incredibly easy, made even easier with 21st-century juice extractors.

I wish you every juicy success and I look forward to hearing your inspirational story soon.

May The Juice Be With You!
Jason the Juice x

1

Juice Yourself Super Slim!

For years I have been aware of the super weight-loss power of freshly extracted juice and good-quality smoothies. However, until I wrote the *7lbs in 7 Days Super Juice Diet*, I didn't realize just how effective they could be in *every* case of overweight and obesity.

The results people were getting were nothing short of remarkable. People weren't simply losing the 7lbs promised, but more like 8lbs, 10lbs and even 14lbs in just 7 days. What's more, they were keeping it off weeks, months and even a year later. Muscle mass *increased*, body fat levels *decreased* and many experienced 'flat stomach enlightenment' in an extremely short amount of time.

7lbs in 7 Days was the first juice-related book ever to hit number one on Amazon and Play.com. At the time it even knocked *The Da Vinci Code* off the top spot. The book has now been translated into many languages and the programme has been used by hundreds of thousands of people including (according to *Now* magazine) Jennifer Aniston, Sarah Jessica Parker, Drew Barrymore and Katie Price (a.k.a. Jordan).

The programme was, and still is, cast-iron proof that an exclusive diet of freshly extracted juice *and* smoothies produces significant *healthy* weight loss. It was a breakthrough by any standards and continues to 'juice' people both mentally and physically in many parts of the world as we speak.

Juice Yourself Slim is, I believe, just as pioneering. This book hasn't been thrown together; a great deal of time, effort, thought and ground-breaking nutritional research has gone into it. It is a programme designed for life. A programme that is so simple, so easy and yet so beautifully effective that anyone can do it without the need for 'dieting' – as you will see. In fact, the programme so easily becomes such a normal part of your daily life that its fat-melting effectiveness is sometimes hard to justify. When you aren't struggling and going round the bend – as is the case on virtually every diet after a period of time – it almost feels like magic or that you have somehow cheated the 'diet' system when you start to look defined and sexy with little or no effort!

This programme is so simple, so easy and yet so beautifully effective that anyone can do it without the need for 'dieting'.

When I devised the programme I knew the results would be good, but given the simplicity and flexibility of *Juice Yourself Slim*, I didn't realize they would be this good. I know you should under-sell and over-deliver, but I am so juiced by this programme I can't lie – the results are mind-blowing. I am genuinely excited for you! I know what you have to look forward to. I know, for example, that you will drop over 7lbs in just the first week, and I know you will have more energy, more spark and feel more juiced about life than you perhaps have in a long time. I know this book will reignite that fire within and I know you will be slimmer *and* healthier as a result. I also know this will be one of the easiest changes of lifestyle you will ever have encountered.

This book deals as much with the mental side of change as the physical, and it's why I am particularly proud to bring this information to you. All you need is an open mind and the conviction to **read every page of this book in the order it was written.** Do that and you will be juicing yourself slim before you know it. However, before we reach that stage we have a lot to get through. First, as you will lose a nice chunk of weight during the first 7 days in particular, I will address an argument which I know will rear its ugly head. An argument usually spouted by a few dieticians and medics who haven't fully grasped the big fat problem.

'But it's Not Good to Lose Weight Quickly!'

You hear this all the time. I heard it a lot when I was interviewed on radio and television about the 7-day juice-only programme. No doubt it's a comment I will get about this new programme too. This advice usually comes from those who aren't fat themselves. Trust me, anyone who is fat is more than happy to drop the pounds in super-fast time. This is why I believe the *7lbs in 7 Days Super Juice Diet* was, and still is, so successful. People saw their fat disappearing before their eyes, and this led to a feeling of momentum and inspiration: two of the most valuable commodities we will ever possess in our quest to emigrate to Slim Land.

Another common remark is 'Quick results often bring quick failures', but it was the super-fast results that *created* the momentum and excitement to continue with a juicy and healthy lifestyle *after* the 7 days. It is because fast results inspire that I have deliberately created a 7-day kick-start part of this lifestyle-changing *Juice Yourself Slim* programme. I believe slow results bring about fast failures. There is, after all, nothing more uninspiring and likely to have you reaching for the cookie jar than losing 1lb a week for a month! At the same time there is nothing more likely to inspire you and keep you motivated than seeing incredible weight loss and at least the outline of what could be a defined stomach in a relatively short space of time.

Juice Yourself to Supreme Health

A point I wish to reiterate over and over again is that this book is not simply about getting slim. Although it is entitled *Juice Yourself Slim*, it could easily have been called 'Juice Yourself to Lower Cholesterol', 'Juice Yourself to Lower Blood Pressure' or 'Juice Yourself to Supreme Health'. However, I know that *some* members of the dietetic and medical professions will be sceptical and disdainful, no matter how extraordinary the improvement in someone's health or weight as a direct result of what they deem an 'alternative' approach.

The World is Flat

In order for dietary and medical breakthroughs to occur, it's essential for the movers and shakers in the health and diet industry to be open to anything that has a fundamentally positive effect on health and obesity, *especially* if it doesn't involve a drug of any kind. If we all still held on to deep-rooted 'facts' written years ago by experts, we would have expanded our world very little due to a fear we would fall off its edge!

As we speak there are hundreds, if not thousands, of 'double blind' tests being carried out by drug companies across the world to find the solution to the Western world's big **FAT** problem. And why wouldn't they? Finding the next licensed 'slimming pill' is big business – sorry, I mean *massive* business – the kind of business that's as corrupt as any other when we are talking big numbers.

Blockbuster: Come and Discover the Financial Difference

Let me give you an idea of what I am talking about here. If a drug company gets their 'fat drug' licensed it is worth well over $1 billion per year. That's **ONE BILLION DOLLARS**. The advertising budget for drugs of this nature can be as much as $150 million (that's apparently more than Pepsi Cola's!). This type of drug is known in the industry as a 'blockbuster', and getting one appears to be the Holy Grail of drug companies. These companies can spend as much as £10,000 trying to convince their main distribution centres – doctors' surgeries – that this new, all-singing, all-dancing drug will solve the world's obesity problem. If they can convince the doctors, they have effectively struck gold, and the pills – no matter how potentially dangerous they are – will be taken by many desperate overweight people. And when you are overweight and it's affecting every aspect of your life, you really can get desperate. We will seemingly try anything, regardless of whether it makes any rational sense or not. I mean, people even thought eggs and bacon swimming around in fat was better for healthy weight loss than fruit after reading the Atkin's Diet. This just shows how our natural intuitive common sense can go out the window when weight loss is promised, and never more so than when weight-loss drugs are involved.

When you are overweight and it's affecting every aspect of your life, you really can get desperate. We will seemingly try anything, regardless of whether it makes any rational sense or not.

There have been many blockbuster 'weight-loss' drugs over the years, each hailed as the new 'wonder' drug. Sometimes, though, I wonder why.

Dying to Lose Weight

Take the 'amazing' weight-loss drug known as phen-phen. So amazing that along with the weight loss came heart disease, hypertension and even death. A lawsuit against phen-phen manufacturer Wyeth found the company responsible for the death of a Texas woman diagnosed with PPH (primary pulmonary hypertension). The woman's family was awarded $1.13 *billion* to compensate for her death due to PPH, caused by taking Pondimin, a phen-phen diet pill. Although this is a rare case, in that the woman actually died, Wyeth have set aside $22 billion to pay damages to over 600,000 people.

Collateral Damage

It has been reported that over 10,000 people in the UK are killed every year by ADRs (adverse drug reactions). To put this in some sort of perspective, there are just over 3,000 people a year killed on our roads in the UK. In the US this figure is estimated at near the 100,000 mark! However, the casualties of ADR are simply viewed as the result of 'friendly fire'. After all, the only reason why 'they' produce such drugs is not to maim or kill but to provide genuine solutions to health problems, especially obesity – a health problem which, coincidentally, just happens to be worth billions for the right pill. What I find incredible is that despite the huge number of undisputed adverse side-effects caused by weight-loss drugs, the argument is always the same: 'They do more good than harm' and 'In the fight against disease and obesity there will inevitably be some casualties until we find the cure.'

The cure, of course, is about as obvious as it gets when it comes to the disease (for that is how it is now classified) known as overweight or obesity. I don't honestly think you need a Harvard degree or a masters in bioscience technology to realize that if someone who is overweight ate less and moved more on a regular basis, they would indeed have found the 'cure'.

However, in reality the 'cure' for overweight and obesity is much more complicated. Genuine addiction to certain foods and drinks plays a *major* part in weight problems, as do a 'diet mentality' and a lack of inspiration. If it were as simple as just knowing what to do to lose weight and keep it off, obesity would be as rare as finding a free parking space in London. Luckily, once you understand how to shift from a 'diet mentality' to one of 'food freedom', as fully described in Chapter 10, then contrary to popular belief, getting slim and *staying* slim can be easy. A full understanding of a 'food freedom' mentality is essential before the brain will even accept that the words 'easy' and 'slimming' can ever go in the same sentence.

Luckily, once you understand how to shift from a 'diet mentality' to one of 'food freedom', then contrary to popular belief, getting slim and staying slim can be easy.

Pharmageddon

It's not just drug companies getting fatter off the fat crisis. There are a million 'alternative' weight-loss remedies out there also searching for their piece of the fat pie. The difference is that when an alternative 'natural' remedy suggests it can help aid weight loss in any way then it is immediately described as 'worthless' and sometimes even 'dangerous' by some of the medical profession. Even today as I write this page there is a headline in the national press which reads:

Herb Cures that Do More Harm than Good

The reason for this bold statement is due to the fact they claim there is 'no scientific evidence' that these therapies work or are safe to use. Dr Canter, who was reported in the *Daily Mail* on 3 October 2007 as saying he wants these treatments banned, said, 'It seems to me if you look at a drug in mainstream medicine it doesn't get used on a patient until its efficacy has been demonstrated.' This same argument seems to be used against just about every type of 'alternative' treatment. But unless I am missing something – or again I've gone mental – haven't there been hundreds, if not thousands, of cases of medical drugs pulled off shelves due to dangerous and sometimes *death-causing* side-effects? Drugs which *were* passed and 'scientifically tested' for 'effectiveness and safety'? Haven't I just talked about what happened with phen-phen?

Then we have the well-publicized Vioxx. This 'scientifically tested drug' was approved yet responsible for tens of thousands of deaths – yes, **TENS OF THOUSANDS!** The drug was designed simply for pain yet was no better than any over-the-counter drug for the same condition. How the hell did this get approval? The answer is simple – **MONEY!** A simple pain-reliever can make billions, so imagine when there's a promise of no more fat – a licence to print money.

Isn't it true that there have been several lawsuits filed against major 'legal' drug companies over fraudulent scientific data? Isn't it also true that the scientific study into a drug's 'effectiveness' and 'safety' is sometimes funded by the producer of the drug itself? Isn't it also true that many of the companies who are responsible for the so-called 'independent' scientific study have a financial interest in the drug company for whom the study is being conducted? In case you didn't know, the shocking answer is *yes*.

Please, if you get nothing else from this book, **DON'T EVER TAKE A WEiGHT-LOSS PiLL.** I hope I can show you in this book that weight loss is within everyone's power. The 'cure' is the same for all and – guess what – it's **NOT** a flipping drug. What a shocker! If you are overweight the cause of your problem is not a 'slimming pill deficiency'. Let's get to the *cause* and quit simply trying to treat the *symptom*.

THE FIRST EVER NON-PRESCRIPTION WEIGHT-LOSS PILL

GlaxoSmithKline launched the 'Alli' pill in the US in 2007. Such is the desperate need for a quick-fix weight loss that 75 million of these drugs were sold in the first six months alone, proving once again that big people are big business for the pharmaceutical industry. By the time you read this book, Alli will probably be on sale in the UK, no prescription needed. Alli often causes oily anal leakage and flatulence if you eat more than their recommended 15g of fat a day.

A Touch of OCD

The main issue I have with any OCD (Over the Counter Drug) weight loss drug is the huge potential for abuse. For people desperate to lose weight, the temptation to take more than the recommended daily dose can be too great. There are many who will wrongly think the more they take the more weight they will lose, and there is no doubt that in some cases people will get obsessed with the drug. It's worth knowing that in the USA Alli sold around $7 million worth of the drug every week (yes, week) at the start of 2008. Not only is there a problem with anal leakage, but Mayo Clinic specialist Donald Hensrud MD estimates Alli

---

would only contribute to about three pounds a year of weight loss. Yes, a year! He also advises users to take a daily multivitamin to help make up for the drug's other negative effect on absorption of fat-soluble vitamins like A, D, E, K and beta carotene.

However, unlike drugs for other diseases, in my view the science behind this drug is flawed for the following reasons, so it's quite easy for people to see that pills are not the solution for fat, and that natural methods are the obvious and only way forward. Alli stops the body absorbing fat in food. This undigested fat, rather than being stored, is passed through the body. This sounds like a dream for most overweight people and no doubt is why millions are buying it. The problem is that these pills can do nothing about the excess refined sugar that is converted into fat. Not only that but **WE NEED FAT!** If these pills get misused (which could easily happen with a non-prescription drug), many could end up with an EFA deficiency. EFA stands for essential fatty acids, the clue here being the word essential. If we don't get a regular supply of good fat we will suffer many adverse health symptoms, which ironically we would no doubt treat with more drugs, keeping the drug merry-go-round going nicely. On top of that, Alli interferes with the absorption of some vitamins, so people are advised to supplement their diet with a daily multivitamin — once again, you really can't make this stuff up! Oh, and the severe diarrhoea which can occur with this drug can also cut the effectiveness of contraceptive pills — brilliant! Once again my advice is as clear as it gets: **NEVER EVER TAKE A WEIGHT-LOSS PILL!**

Fat Lies

There have been many cases of 'foods' that have passed every test in the book for human consumption which have proved years later to be extremely harmful. Take trans-fats for just one of hundreds of possible examples. A recent report from the Food Standards Agency (FSA) said, 'The trans-fats found in food containing hydrogenated vegetable oil are harmful and have no known nutritional benefits. They raise the type of cholesterol in the blood that increases the risk of coronary heart disease. Some evidence suggests that the effects of these trans-fats may be worse than saturated fats.'

The question I have is a simple one: how come this wasn't known *before* this type of fat entered the food chain? Why, after all the 'tests' and 'research' which is required before any food is passed, weren't the harmful effects spotted? One thing's for sure: if this type of adverse reaction was ever seen with any type of juice therapy it would be banned *immediately*, and no doubt I would be up on some kind of charge for 'endangering the health of others' and possibly even 'manslaughter'. What's mental is that despite the fact these harmful effects of trans-fats are known and have been known for over 20 years, there is still (at the time of writing) no obligation for food manufacturers to display the amount of trans-fats on product labels.

EGG ON HER FACE

In 1988 a senior government scientist became convinced that a general rise in salmonella poisoning in the UK must be caused by the bacteria getting inside chickens' eggs. The junior health minister at the time – Edwina Currie – took his comments on board and made a public announcement which led to complete panic. Millions of chickens were slaughtered and thousands of small egg producers were put out of business. Four years later the government reversed its policy, acknowledging that eggs had not been the problem after all. Just one scientist's opinion gets taken as read and millions suffer.

The point I am making is that just because something has been 'medically and/or scientifically tested' for 'effectiveness and safety', it doesn't necessarily mean it is effective or in any way safe. And, again, it isn't true to say drugs are always *fully tested for their safety and effectiveness* before going into the public domain – just read Dr Richard Halvorsen's superb book *The Truth About Vaccines* with regard to the short time the MMR jab was 'tested' before being made almost compulsory.

If all the medicines that were tested were super effective there wouldn't be a multi-billion-dollar alternative market. After all, we all pay into the kitty and life would be much cheaper if most medical treatment had the 'good and positive' effect so often claimed. When I was covered from head to foot in psoriasis the only treatment I was offered at the time was either high-potency steroid cream or going to hospital and being covered in 'tar' and bandages for six weeks. Both treatments would have 'thinned' my skin and caused me to become sensitive to sunlight, which, ironically, is one of the best natural treatments for this skin condition. Both treatments would also have done nothing whatsoever to try to get to the cause of problem.

In countries such as Denmark, people with severe skin conditions such as psoriasis are flown to the Dead Sea in Israel for one month in order to treat their condition. The enlightened medical profession, along with those responsible for the best use of taxpayers' money, realized that it actually costs less to send patients to the Dead Sea for a month than it does to keep them in hospital covered in bandages for six weeks. Not only is it better value for money but it is extremely effective as well. The Dead Sea is one of the most unique places on earth, highly dense in natural healing salts and minerals, as well as being the lowest place on earth – making it one of the safest places to get natural sunlight therapy. I was *never* offered this option, and despite what I put into the 'kitty', I always had to pay my own way to Israel, as well as for any alternative treatment for my condition. It is nice to know that we all pay for health care many times over, once in tax and once again in 'alternative' measures *when*, not so much *if*, any 'tested' medical treatment fails us.

PATENTLY Obvious

It seems odd to me that natural fruit and plant remedies (such as pure juice therapy), which have been responsible for zero direct deaths, are often hammered by the medical profession, yet medical weight-loss drugs which often do cause harm are all considered part of the 'friendly fire' syndrome. That isn't to say that the medical profession doesn't often have a very valid point. Some of the weight-loss products out there are about as effective as a cat flap in an elephant house and a total waste of time and money, and yes, there are unscrupulous characters in every business. But the same argument can often be levelled at medical drugs for weight loss.

In fact, I don't know of one single weight-loss drug that has come even close to solving the obesity epidemic anywhere in the world. Despite this I can guarantee it won't be long before you read about the next 'amazing breakthrough in weight loss' drug therapy (look in your newspaper today, it may be there). This drug will come with a clean bill of health and backed by studies of many who have lost X amount of weight because of the drug. Once again, if you do ever see the new answer to everyone's fat problem wrapped up in a drug pill DON'T TAKE IT (just in case you missed that earlier!). All drugs have side-effects and all drugs are toxic to the body. If you are already taking a weight-loss pill, talk to your GP before you decide to stop taking it. I have to say that, but the same piece of advice would never apply to anything healthy. I doubt you'll ever hear: 'Before you stop eating avocados check with your GP first' – why? Because fruit and vegetables aren't dangerous and don't cause withdrawal symptoms of any kind.

Fat People = Fat Profits

The reason for the apparent 'new' weight-loss drugs is not out of a genuine care for our health, which would be nice. In 1998, GPs in the UK spent just £20,000 on anti-obesity drugs yet in 2005 the annual cost had risen to more than £38 million. That's one hell of a big fat jump. Why such a jump? Simple. Obesity has now been reclassified as a disease. Why does this make such a difference? Again, simple. As a disease it needs to be treated, and as a disease – in the minds of the 'professionals' and indeed aspects of the law – this means an increase in medical 'help'. And medical help, of course, equals drugs! Drugs for weight loss in particular equal mega profits, more disease and more toxicity.

It's worth knowing that in the US the FDA (Food and Drug Administration) passed a law stating, **'only a drug can cure, prevent, or treat a disease'.** The law is exactly the same in the UK. In 1996 a ruling was made that anyone making a claim that any food can cure, prevent or treat a disease is breaking the law and is subject to criminal prosecution. This effectively means that if someone were to say that fruit can help to prevent cancer or obesity, they could go to jail for it! This is why when a major UK supermarket stated that mangos could help in the prevention of certain cancers, they were brought to book and it made national news. The 'offending' sign was removed. But mangos *do* help with the prevention of disease, as do apples, pears, oranges, lemons, spinach and ALL other fruits and vegetables designed for human consumption. All contain antioxidants and all help to curb free radical damage, which even by the government's own admission is one of the biggest causes of disease and premature aging.

Listen carefully to what I am saying here as it beggars belief on every level. There is a law that effectively says there will never be a *natural* remedy that can cure, prevent or treat a disease. No one will ever be able to make such a claim, even if it's 100 per cent true. How mind-blowingly absurd is that? It means that if someone advertised that oranges or lemons could cure the killer disease 'scurvy' (which, of course, they do and this is not disputed by anyone), they could be thrown into jail. No, I am not joking, but I sincerely wish I were. For if oranges or lemons were deemed to cure, prevent or treat the disease scurvy, they would then be classed as 'drugs'. However, before a 'drug' label can be given, these fruits would have to go through the £400,000 worth of testing required to approve a new drug. This would never happen. Why? Well, a natural remedy cannot be patented by anyone and so who on earth would ever pay that amount of money for testing if they couldn't get that money back at least tenfold? You see, it's not always about actually curing, preventing or genuinely treating disease; it's all about what can be patented. If it can't – forget it. If it can – bingo!

Let's not forget that if fruit and vegetables were claimed to cure, treat or prevent a new disease like 'obesity', then anyone selling them without a licence to dispense medicine would be prosecuted. Yes, if someone were to state that a lemon was a cure for scurvy, or that avocados were a good treatment for obesity, the lemon suddenly stops being a lemon and the avocado stops being an avocado. They both now miraculously become drugs – yes, a lemon a drug. And unless you have a licensed practice or sell medicine, you could be nicked! Once again, you really can't make this stuff up.

Obesity, now it's a disease, is mega business for the medical drug industry. And the more people who are diagnosed with obesity, the fatter the nation looks and the fatter the profits. It's worth knowing that obesity is diagnosed using a very antiquated system called the BMI index. BMI stands for body mass index. It is a measurement of fat which is worked out by taking your weight in kilograms and dividing it by your height in metres. What it doesn't take into account is body muscle weight. This means that Brad Pitt, according to the BMI index, is obese – yes, Brad Pitt obese! This should illustrate perfectly what a stupid system this is. But if it means more people are diagnosed with obesity, even if in the real world they aren't obese, all the better for the new drug on the block.

The Sicker We Get, the Healthier Their Profits

The fact of the matter is there will never be a drug that will enable the body to lose weight in a natural and *healthy* way. ALL drugs have negative side-effects, and these side-effects are very often treated with more drugs. Unless people get ill, drugs become worthless. Drugs often create the need simply for more drugs, and more drugs mean more profit. The big drug companies are PLCs, and as public limited companies they have to, **BY LAW,** *increase* profits for their shareholders. How can you have a situation where the people responsible for drug treatments being dispensed to the public are lawfully obliged to increase profits? How can this be when increased profits can *only* occur if more people take more drugs? Drugs which, let's not forget, have adverse side-effects. Side-effects which, let's not forget, are responsible for over 10,000 deaths in the UK alone each year. This is like putting traffic wardens on performance pay and giving them bonuses if they hand out more parking tickets, a system which would inevitably lead to corruption and the removal of common sense – oh sorry, this is the system!

Money Makes the Drug World Go Round and Round and Round

Weight-loss drugs are the new blockbusters on the pharmaceutical block. They will increasingly rear their ugly heads and all in the name of 'help'. The problem is the only people these drugs tend to help are the shareholders and directors of the big pharmaceutical companies.

The reality is that the powerful nutritious liquid fuel trapped within the fibres of raw fruits and vegetables contains the perfect balance of vitamins, minerals, fats, carbohydrates and amino acids to maintain health during weight loss. There are some who will be arrogant enough to think they can create something more perfect than nature itself to deal with the obesity nightmare taking place in our world at this time, but I hope and feel that common sense and intuition will have the majority of people going in the right direction.

You Can't Patent Fruit or Veg

Once again, the biggest problem is that you cannot patent a fruit or vegetable. No patent means no big blockbuster money-spinner. What I find most extraordinary is how no one seems to question what many scientists in this field are doing. They often do a study and find that a certain fruit or vegetable is highly effective for either the prevention or treatment of a particular disease. They then try to find exactly which ingredient contained within the fruit or vegetable makes it so effective. Their aim, I imagine, is to isolate the secret ingredient and add some other chemicals to it in order to make a patentable 'drug'. A 'drug' which will once again be hailed as the new all-singing, all-dancing answer to whatever disease the fruit or vegetable helped with. Just a thought here, but why on earth don't they simply suggest people eat the fruit or vegetable that made the difference? Is it really because you can't patent it? Could the industry be that corrupt?

'Lies, damn lies and statistics.'

— Mark Twain

You can make any study look and sound better than it actually is, especially when you are trying to get a licence for a blockbuster drug. Not all studies are worthless, clearly, and many are extremely valid. However, as far as I'm concerned there is only one study worth looking at and that is genuine people giving genuine testimonials. We live in a world where if people say a drug has helped them in any way it is taken as read by the medical profession, but if a load of people get spectacular results for their health or ailment using natural methods, the usual responses are: 'it hasn't been tested properly' and 'it might have worked for those people, but there is no evidence to suggest it will work for everyone'. But there's no evidence to suggest any drug on earth will work for everyone either. There is also no evidence to suggest we are making any progress whatsoever with 'drug therapy' for weight loss in any part of the world, yet many millions are still being invested into finding *the* cure-all 'anti-obesity pill'.

True Scientific Success

I have received thousands of genuine emails from people all over the world who have had *major* health problems massively reduced or eliminated as a direct result of freshly extracted juice and nutritious freshly made smoothies. There will also be countless people who have had diseases prevented due to getting into a juicy and healthier lifestyle, the extent of which we will never know.

What I find shocking is that instead of many people in the dietetic and medical professions looking into this as a potential breakthrough natural treatment for obesity and other ailments, we have a situation where my programmes, such as *7lbs in 7 Days*, are attacked instead of embraced. When you read the results in the next chapter, you will be blown away and will think it even more of a mystery why freshly extracted juice as a therapy isn't embraced more widely.

'The drugs don't work.'

— The Verve

It often takes years for some dieticians and the mass medical profession to catch up and accept any alternative to drug treatment. We are only now getting doctors and dieticians recommending things like fish oil for joint pain, even though this has been spouted by the non-medical clan for decades. Even as I write, I have just heard the news on the BBC headlining the result of a scientific study showing how a cocktail of additives can cause hyperactivity in some children – something which, once again, the 'alternative' voice of common sense has been saying for donkey's years. When you see bright green, often luminous drinks masquerading as 'juice', containing a chemical concoction any science academy would be proud of, I don't think you need six years of medical training to instinctively know it just might send your kids nuts!

What has happened to common sense? What has happened to that inner knowing we all possess? Things become even more insane when you think that some of the top-selling children's medicines contain some of these hyperactive-causing chemicals, as well as other lovely things such as aspartame. Aspartame is an artificial sweetener which has been linked to 92 different harmful side-effects, including brain tumours. You can't make this stuff up.

'Anti-wrinkle cream there may be but anti-fat bastard cream there certainly is not.'

— from the film THE FULL MONTY

We are, despite what some are saying, in the grip of a genuine obesity and overweight epidemic. This isn't *Daily Mail* headline stuff either. It's common knowledge to most in the know and blatantly obvious to all who walk down Walsall High Street on a Saturday afternoon! It has been reported that if current trends continue, 50 per cent of all children in the UK will be significantly overweight or obese by the year 2050. It won't be long before we are on a par with the US, where at the time of writing a whopping **two-thirds of US citizens are overweight or obese.** That's two-thirds! Along with being overweight and obese comes diabetes, heart disease, stroke, cancer, gout, arthritis, high blood pressure, high LDL cholesterol levels, hyperactive disorder and so the list goes on and on.

Everything we put into our system changes our biochemistry, and given that blood flows through the brain there is no question that many mental disorders are also caused by a lack of nutrients and the addition of clogging 'foods' and 'drinks'. Even the World Heath Organization recognizes that 85 per cent of all disease is a direct result of what we put into our mouths and external environmental factors, such as living in a polluted city.

'i am too chubby, too large ... it's not good!'

— Luciano Pavarotti

Being overweight is often an addictive and uninspired trap. As it has a knock-on effect on the manifestation of virtually all of mankind's common and debilitating diseases, it really is something we should be paying full attention to. This is why it is of paramount importance that the mainstream dietetic and medical world gets on board with any treatment that is clearly effective in this area. Juicing is not only super effective, but it's also safe, healthy and something people can do every day of their lives with *no* adverse side-effects whatsoever. If a drug was produced that had the same effect, it would be hailed as the new obesity and disease 'wonder' drug, and every doctor and dietician would be singing its praises and prescribing it left, right and centre.

Juicing is not only super effective, but it's also safe, healthy and something people can do every day of their lives with NO adverse side-effects whatsoever.

Being overweight, as I know from my past, is no picnic. People who have never suffered are the first to simply say, 'Eat less and move more.' This sounds logical and obvious, and who can blame them for saying such a thing. However, logic plays no part in addiction. It's like saying to a smoker, 'Smoking is bad and if you stopped you'd have more money and would be healthier.' That kind of statement might be correct, but it's somewhat patronizing to think the smoker has no idea of these obvious facts.

It is just as patronizing to inform someone who is overweight that, 'If you eat more good stuff, cut down on rubbish and exercise more you will be slimmer and feel better.' When I was overweight and I heard people saying this to me I would simply think, 'No shit, Sherlock!' Just because someone is thick physically it doesn't automatically make them thick mentally. I was fully aware of what I was doing. I had lost my fire, my inspiration – that impetus which makes us want to bounce out of bed and embrace the opportunities life has to offer. I had simply lost my spark, something that happens to so many people on a regular basis.

'My dream is to wake up 50lbs less and fly.'

— Luciano Pavarotti

Luckily, times really are changing. Increasing numbers of doctors and dieticians are realizing that drugs don't work when it comes to weight loss. Many are also more open-minded than ever when it comes to possible new options. Even the resident Radio 2 doctor – Dr Jarvis – often recommends cognitive therapy for many ailments, including obesity. This is why this book, like all of my others, deals with the mental as much as the physical. Things are changing so much that I even have many doctors who recommend my books and work, but I feel we are some time off mainstream medical heads being as open. I also feel it will be many more years before 'juice therapy' of any kind is recognized as an extremely safe and effective treatment for obesity and other disease.

I wish to make something clear at this point: I am all for medical intervention and drugs where necessary. I *strongly* believe I wouldn't be alive today without the injection which saved my life when I had my very first asthma attack at the age of eight. However, I wish I had been told what was *causing* my condition instead of simply being given drugs for the next God knows how many years to sticky tape over the root cause of the problem. It would have been good if someone had at least suggested that diet and exercise just *might* play a part. At least then I could have tried to do something about it instead of just accepting my drug-filled days. However, as I will keep saying, there's a lot of money in drugs – more than most of us can comprehend – so what interest has a drug company got in actually curing your condition? Just a thought.

Pure Common Sense Science

Science, as far as I am concerned, is 'that which works'. For obesity and weight loss there is no question – juicing works! Exercise works! It not only works for some; it works for *everyone* – and I am willing to challenge anyone who believes anything to the contrary. This means that no matter what you have tried before, the *physical* weight-loss results are guaranteed on this programme.

However, this book isn't simply about the physical. It's also about igniting that inspirational mental fire within – that passion, which often sits dormant inside us all. When ignited, it makes us feel anything is possible. It makes us excited about life again, and makes us *want* to get up, exercise and get slim so we can get the most out of each and every day.

As mentioned in the Introduction, many people think that life has put out the fire. While we are breathing, however, it is a sure sign that the pilot light is very much on, and all that's required is a bit of mental fuel to ignite the fire once again. What we don't realize is that there are many aspects that dampen the fire. There are many 'foods', for example, that contain toxic chemicals which gradually wear us down without our knowledge. We often take over-the-counter drugs to deal with some of the nutritional deficiencies caused by these 'foods'. These drugs **ALL** have negative side-effects, which once again contribute to the dampening of our inspirational fires.

There are many things that can ignite us once again. Sometimes it can be just a sentence. For others it's hearing of other people's successes. It can be seeing what you deem 'real' scientific studies on juicing. It can be seeing the truth behind the food companies and deciding you no longer want to help fund them by passing over your hard-earned money in exchange for substances which will simply make you fat, ill and unhappy. Whatever it is, this book has been carefully designed to ignite that fire within and give you a successful launch on your juicy journey to the lovely world of slimness and health.

Nothing, I feel, can trigger the pilot light to fire more so than people who have already experienced incredible success. When you see what can be achieved in a short space of time, it helps to start the firing process. I have chosen just a tiny selection from our juicy postbag to help light that juicy fire within. Make a point of reading every one, as some of the results will astound you. I also sincerely hope that those sceptics in the dietetic and medical worlds read the next chapter and take note. I hope it makes them sit up, pay attention and start to see the incredible value freshly extracted juice can have on every aspect of mental and physical health. I also hope they, and you for that matter, don't dismiss these letters and emails as 'isolated' or 'not real'. The following are all *100 per cent genuine*, from 'real' people from every walk of life. All have different lifestyles, jobs, commitments, ages, and yet all managed to introduce juicing into their often hectic lives and reap the slimming and health rewards. Come forth and let me give you a glimpse of what can happen when you join in …

2

The Juice Revolution

There is a juice revolution happening and people of all ages and from all walks of life are seeing and feeling the results. Even Victoria Beckham and Kate Moss have been reported to have been at the wheatgrass shots!

Juicing is no longer seen as something for mad people with long hair who spend much of their lives in trees protesting against a new bypass being built. Today, juicing and smoothie-making is viewed as a genuine and highly effective way to get better health and a super-slim body. A little over five years ago, less than 1 per cent of the UK population owned a juice extractor; that figure is now 6 per cent and is expected to reach 20 per cent by the year 2012. Not only are people buying them, but unlike gadgets like bread-makers, they are even starting to use them – what a concept!

Today, juicing and smoothie-making is viewed as a genuine and highly effective way to get better health and a super-slim body.

This chapter is dedicated to illustrating the truly amazing health and slimming results that can be achieved by incorporating **freshly extracted** fruit and vegetable juices into your life. You can have all the scientific studies in the world, but none will get your juices flowing more than the remarkable results of others.

I have heard some amazing stories over the years and have seen at first hand some truly wonderful and almost miraculous changes. I have seen people come off antidepressants after years of taking them. I have seen people with arthritis who could barely move climb a steep hill and walk miles after incorporating juicing into their lives. I have seen skin disorders virtually disappear as well, of course, as excess fat seemingly melt away.

In a recent seminar I conducted, an 80-year-old man asked a question: 'What are you supposed to do if your partner thinks you're insane for juicing?' I suggested that if he were told by a doctor that he should be taking something like a statin drug for high cholesterol she would *insist* he took them, so she should be as understanding when he is trying to treat his health with something natural. His reply was perhaps one of the most priceless I have ever heard: 'Oh that's the other thing. I am meant to be on a statin for high cholesterol, but since I have been juicing I have no need … but we're having to keep that one a secret – don't tell the wife!'

It would be almost impossible to read this chapter without it adding at least a few flames to your fire. Inspiration is such a vital catalyst to any kind of change, especially when you are trying to kick-start a healthy eating and slimming plan. And there is nothing more inspirational or motivating than seeing real results.

Here are just a few of the hundreds of thousands of genuine emails I have received over the years. I have made comments after some of them to fully illustrate some of the points. I would like to thank the thousands of people who have taken the time to write to me. Even if it takes a few months I always make a point of reading and replying to as many as possible. It was hard to pick out just a few. However, I hope this small selection enables you to see the sort of health and slimming magic that can occur with the help of the right frame of mind, a few fruits and vegetables, a juicer and a blender.

Please do not make the mistake of skipping the letters. They all have a message and they all help to lay the foundations. Remember, everything I have written is for a reason; every word has a point to it; and every one of the letters you read here is 100 per cent genuine and unsolicited. The magic is in their words – don't miss them.

❝ Subject: Yippee! i never have to go on another diet!!!

WOW! Where do i start? Since having two kids 13 and 10 years ago my weight has gone up and down like you wouldn't believe. Like many people i've done The Cabbage Soup Diet and Weight Watchers (brill, no more counting those bloody points!) to name but a few, but it wasn't until September of last year that i found that juicing really and truly works for me. it really has been amazing — life-changing in fact. (i know you most probably hear this all the time!)

i have since lost 2 stone. i have gone from 11st 4lbs to 9st 3lbs. Size 14 to size 10. in fact, i am wearing a size 8 top at the moment … i haven't done that for years! One of the reasons i am emailing you is that the friends i have introduced juicing to keep saying 'you must tell him how well you've done' or 'you should be one of his reps'. i know you've had an email this week from Louise who's done really well. She's just one of the people i've introduced it to. My neighbour Maria has lost 9lbs in one week and my husband is doing it at the moment and has lost 6lbs since Monday (he was a bit sceptical at first). i'm sooo proud of all of them. i think to date it's well over 4 stone between us all. Also, my kids love the smoothies. it just feels so good to see them drink all that live goodness.

i must admit that when we go on holiday i get really crabby because i can't do my juicing. Of course i always choose the healthy option now, which isn't too bad. in fact, when i see people sitting in places like McDonald's i feel sorry for them when they could quite easily go somewhere else and have something healthier. i have turned into a bit of the Food Police, and when my kids see something that's not very nice they go 'Oooh that's toxic!' Well at least it's got them thinking about what they are putting in their mouths. Louise and i are coming to your seminar in Manchester, which we are really excited about, and i'm saving like mad to go on one of your Ultimate Retreat weeks next year.

Well you've most probably had enough of my waffling now so as a last note i just want to say THANK YOU. You really have changed our lives, for which i will be eternally grateful.

Many thanks
Paula '

The weight loss is one thing but what interested me most was the knock-on effect success like this has. Not only has Paula lost over 28lbs and a few dress sizes, but because of her success her neighbour did it and lost 9lbs in one week, and even Paula's husband who was a sceptic lost 6lbs in just a few days. What is also wonderful is how this kind of influence has an effect on their children too. Juicing and smoothie-making creates theatre in the kitchen and kids are often mesmerized by it.

' Hi Jason and team
Just wanted you to know i recently bought a juicer from you and am now mad on it! Lost a stone in weight in just under three weeks! And that was not really why i started. i had headaches most evenings, hay fever and allergies. Anyway, my headaches have gone and so has everything else. i feel great, and i'm not actually going mad on my intake, just one or two juices a day with a healthy meal. So far i've converted three other people because of the way i now look!

i'm so pleased i listen to Steve Wright on Radio 2 as that's where i heard about this. Cheers Jason — Happy Juicing

M. Waller '

Headaches gone, hay fever gone and 14lbs lighter in under three weeks without even trying. Just by having a couple of juices and smoothies a day with a healthy meal – which, funnily enough, is exactly the principle of the *Juice Yourself Slim* programme. Once again, they have converted three of their friends because of the way they now look – the juice revolution is happening!

> **Dear Mr Vale**
> My husband and i are very much enjoying drinking delicious juices as a result of reading your books. Not only do we have more energy and better health but our hair is also going back to its original colour! We are 68 and 73 years old, so that is a wonderful surprise!
>
> **Yours sincerely**
> **Audrey S**

What's wonderful about this email isn't so much that their hair started to go back to its original colour (although **WOW!**) but that at 68 and 73 years old they are willing to try new things in the 21st century health world. They're not alone either. I am receiving more and more letters and emails from people in, let's say, the mature part of their life. The digestive system often gets weak as the years go on, and juicing and smoothie-making are the perfect way to get 'live' nutrients into a weak system. I honestly can't wait till I get our juice and smoothie bars up and running in hospitals. If there was ever a place crying out for excellent nutrition that's easy to digest and assimilate, it's hospitals.

> **i have got so much energy and mental clarity ... and i am so happy because i have got my 90-year-old grandad into juicing and he loves it!**

Once again proving the fact it's never too late to teach an old dog new juicy tricks!

'Hi Jason

i would just like to say thank you so much! i'm 15 and have been
overweight all my life, constantly trying to slim down. That was
until my mum bought your book and i read it. i've lost a stone
and the weight just keeps going. i've never been happier or felt
better. Thank you!

Jenny'

Here's someone at the other end of the age spectrum. Jenny is just 15 years old – the book clearly inspired her and the juices were the exact fuel required to catapult her to change, something she had been trying to do for years. I have had hundreds, if not thousands, of emails from people of 16 years of age or less. I remember one particular boy aged just 12 who lost over 3 stone after reading *Slim 4 Life*. The weight loss is one thing, but to read a book of this nature at just 12 years old is I feel a feat in itself. I know many adults who buy these books but never actually read them.

We live in a weight-obsessed society and one thing is for sure: teenage girls (and boys) will often follow just about anything their idol is doing to look great, no matter how bats it may be. To give you an example, after Victoria Beckham was seen reading a particular weight-loss book aimed mainly at teenagers entitled *Skinny Bitch*, sales increased by 4,000 per cent that same day! If a celebrity a teenager looks up to decides to drink oil and eat leather to lose weight, they will follow. One of the many good things which came from Jordan doing the juicing pro-gramme was the tremendous influence she had on teenage girls look-ing to lose weight. Teenagers up and down the country started juicing fresh celery, cucumber, pineapple, apple, lime and spinach and blend-ing it with avocado and ice to make the now famous Turbo Charge Smoothie – the very one Jordan was having daily. Tweenagers (ages 8–12) and teenagers drinking vegetables! A breakthrough by any stan-dards, I'm sure you'll agree.

'Just had to share my delight with you … i have lost 18lbs in 14 days! Truly amazing as i have tried them all before and never had such startling results with such ease and enjoyment. My husband looks and feels 10 years younger and is even spreading the word to his 'food police' mates. i overheard him explaining to one that 'it isn't a diet, it's a permanent change of lifestyle'. i was so proud!! Thank you, thank you, thank you. i am now going to order some more books and CDs for friends who need them. Another disciple is born!

Alison'

I already hear cries from anyone reading this from the dietetic or medical world of 'that's far too much weight in such a short space of time' along with 'it's not healthy to do such a thing' and so on. However, I can also hear at the same time the cries of people who suffer from obesity: 'WOW – now that's the kind of results I can get on board with!'

We all know that this woman didn't lose 18lbs of fat and that of course a great deal of the weight loss must have been water, but so what? This kind of weight loss has given her the one commodity essential to good health and continued weight loss – **momentum**. If she had been on a normal 'steady weight-loss' plan and lost only, say, 1–2lbs, she would have felt deflated, and the chances of her continuing would have been slim, unlike herself. However, such drastic weight loss has lifted her spirits; it has ignited that elusive fire within and launched her to change. I agree that if this kind of weight loss is achieved by chemical liquid shakes or pure fasting (where a person has no nutrition whatsoever) then I would be joining the 'it's not healthy gang', but as it was achieved by drinking the finest freshly extracted juices, it's hard to find an argument against it.

‘Hi Jason and the Juicy Team

i am sure you must be inundated with emails of thanks but this one is really sincere and from the heart. i am somewhat confused by the fact that in the past six weeks i have lost 14 pounds and am now the same size i was 12 years ago. i found your book in a juice bar in Bath, having never heard of you before. Yes, i had heard of Jordan and vaguely remember when she started juicing but did not really take that much interest — in my view she looked fabulous before juicing and was naturally skinny and would have bounced back anyway after having her baby. i WAS WRONG!

i have tried every silly diet going and the only weight i ever lost was just a few pounds which i put straight back on. My poor husband watched me suffer and boy was i bad tempered during these fads. This time he watched with great interest. i gave up alcohol easily. i gave up sugar and chocolate very easily (big shock as i am major addict). i even started working out twice a day and enjoyed it. He could not resist — he joined me on it and has lost 12 pounds so far in about four weeks. We would love to comment in anything you publish on how great this has been for us if you ever need extra testimonials. i am sure you have thousands but it's good to feel we can give you something back.

it must drive you nuts, trying to get people to just do what you say and let the magic happen. i feel that you have given me a special secret of health, wellbeing and a longer life. You have also saved me a fortune as i now fit back into all my fabulous clothes. So for that i thank you (which seems like two very small words compared to what you have done for us).

This Christmas i have sent your books to family and friends. i am very happy to pass this gift to others who are in need.

You are an angel — thank you ... thank you ... thank you.
Annie **’**

One comment here is perhaps more poignant than any other: '… do what you say and let the magic happen'. And I can't think of a better word than 'magic' to describe what happens when you start to give your body the finest liquid fuel and stop putting in rubbish. Many of the stories I read can only be described as miraculous, and I guess we should never underestimate the power of nature, its natural ability to heal and inherent desire to keep us alive.

‘ i would like to say thank you so very much as i've just done the plan and am overwhelmed with joy. i started out weighing in at 12st 7lbs, and today is the eighth day and i now weigh 11st 12lbs. i am 37 years old and i haven't weighed 11st anything for 10 years. My body fat was 36.7, now it's 33.3. Water was 46.0, now 48.2. Muscle mass was 32.0, now 33.5. BMi was 28.3, now 26.8, and basal was 1561, now 1520. i am gobsmacked.

i loved all the juices except the pure green super juice. Like you said, i only had three or four juices a day because i wasn't hungry. i have had a juicer for a while now and got stuck in the rut of making the same juice every day, but now i look forward to getting all my ingredients out ready to juice. i've read the turbo charge book so that's going to help no end in my next step in life, and then i'm going out shopping for new clothes. Ha ha! i can't thank you enough, Jason.

A couple of years ago i weighed 15st 1lb so i joined Weight Watchers. in the beginning it was good and right for me but as time went on i found i got sick of constantly working out how many points was in every single thing i put into my mouth. i felt as though it had taken over my life and i had stopped losing weight so i left. if they could see me now, ha ha! Well, here's to forever. i love my new self and new life. i've dug out my old bike and used it no end and i've been bouncing for England, so once again thank you all.

Love
P Ward ’

Please take a moment to look at the stats. Yes, she has lost 9lbs in the seven days, but more importantly, look at the muscle mass and body fat. Before, the muscle mass was 32 and is now 33.5, and the body fat was 36.7 and is now 33.3 just seven days later. One of the first things anyone in the dietetic or medical profession says about my juice programme (before they test it at all) is that if a person were to live on nothing but juice for one week then all they would lose is muscle and water and very little, if any, actual fat. However, time after time I get emails with stats like these – muscle INCREASES and fat DECREASES.

‘ Hi to Jason and everyone — wanted to say THANKS.
i bought a juicer last week and got the book free with it. i decided to only replace two main meals per day and have rice and veg, fish or tofu, stir-fried or steamed, in the evening.
　FOR THE FIRST TIME IN YEARS i FEEL FANTASTIC!!!!
　i HAVE ENERGY! IT'S WONDERFUL.
　i was drinking far too much alcohol although my food was healthy with plenty of fresh fruit, veg and grains. But Monday of last week i decided that i had to do something as my weight was just going up and up — i am 53 and 5 feet tall and the scales were threatening to go over the 11st mark. i felt terrible and had scalp problems which wouldn't heal after becoming intolerant to hair dye last September.
　The JUICES are DELICIOUS!!! and so easy. After a week i have lost 4lbs, my scalp is healing and i even ran down the road with my grandchildren on Monday!
　So again, thank you. i love fruit and veg anyway but these cocktails are so tasty. i am already experimenting with different ingredients as i really enjoy fresh food. i'm gradually weaning my husband on to juices as well.

Thanks again ’

For the first time in years this 53-year-old women feels fantastic and more energetic. She's lost weight and her scalp is healing – again, all in the short space of just seven days. All she has done is introduce a couple of juices a day into her life and eat an evening meal – once again, *exactly* the principles of *Juice Yourself Slim*. She lost 4lbs without even trying, which is the beauty of this programme. As well as being highly effective – it's easy! As you will discover soon.

‘**Dear Jason**

On Sunday (day 19 on the juice trial) i did the 10K Bananaman Chase. i took your advice and had a banana with my juice in the morning and i was really nervous. i knew i would do it but thought it would take me a lot longer than my last 10K at the beginning of September … Well, anyway, i am so proud of myself because i have just had the official timing for the race on Sunday and i have knocked six minutes off my last run. Yippee! i was literally RUNNiNG ON JUiCE. X

Annette’

Annette was one of the people on the Super Juice Me! test programme. The small group lived on only juice and smoothies for 30 days. Annette was on day 19 of this programme when she decided to run the 10K race. As you can see, she not only completed the race but knocked six minutes off her previous time. We have been conditioned to believe we need to load up on complex carbohydrates before any kind of distance running, but time and time again I have seen people literally 'running on juice'. When I was on day five of a juice-only programme I ran a half marathon, and I completed the New York full marathon with just a couple of Super Fuel Smoothies in me (*see page 218*). This woman had been living on nothing but juice and smoothies for 19 days before the race, and far from collapsing, she sailed home. Never underestimate the carbohydrate and 'isotonic' powers of freshly extracted juice!

ᶜDear Juice Master Team

i accidentally stumbled on Jason's book when i purchased my new juicer from John Lewis. My first reaction was to bin the book because at 5' 6" and 8st in weight i had no desire or need to lose weight. i read the first few pages and persevered as the book had asked me to and then became interested in the nutritional aspects.

i proceeded to give juicing a shot just for the hell of it. Things then started happening quite quickly even though i was not doing the juicing diet itself but just taking two or three juices a day on a regular basis. The first thing was that my system flushed out. Then i had more energy and felt like exercising more and sleeping less. Finally, within a period of three months, my endometriosis disappeared quite unexpectedly after eight years, several miscarriages and numerous treatments.

So thank you!
Regards
Tayba ˈ

You would think after reading such a letter that anyone in the medical or dietetic industry would want to know more. After all, if eight years of *numerous* medical treatments have failed and only three months of juicing has seen the condition 'completely disappear', surely someone, somewhere who can make a bigger difference than me, should at least look into it with an open mind. What shouldn't happen is what so often does: it gets dismissed as pseudo-science.

Endometriosis is a condition affecting some two million women in the UK alone. It can cause pain, swelling and bleeding, and can occur in many parts of the body, most commonly the fallopian tubes, ovaries, bladder, bowel, intestines and vagina. So what's the usual approach to treatment? Anything from simple anti-inflammatory drugs to surgery. Side-effects of some of the drug treatments used for this condition include bloating, mood changes, irregular bleeding, acne, **weight gain** and even the development of masculine features (hair growth and deepening voice). So your endometriosis might get better but you may well be walking around with the voice of Darth Vader, the face of Wolf Boy and a stomach the size of the Napa Valley!

The side-effects from the 'alternative' juicing approach were simply more energy and less sleep. Doesn't it seem odd that when what is deemed an 'alternative' approach works, it is viewed by many as meaningless, but if a drug has the slightest positive effect it's on the shelves quicker than you can say 'blockbuster'.

❛Hello there

i just wanted to thank Jason … about a million times over really. i started juicing a while back as i bought a juicer and it came with one of Jason's books. i have always tried to watch what i eat but reading this book was very helpful in getting me to juice every evening after work.

Since 16 June, i have lost about a stone and a half and feel amazing. i promote Jason and his book and the health benefits wherever i go, and people are amazed when they taste how good the juices can be. it's now part of my life and i don't want to go back to former eating patterns. At 5' 2" i have always struggled with my weight but juicing has made steady weight loss EASY. i have a healthy meal in the evening which mostly consists of an enormous salad with something else (have always been nuts about salads anyway). Everyone is telling me how good i look and although i still have a little way to go to be a perfect weight (if there is such a thing) i am relaxed about getting there.

i feel like i've got a whole new set of clothes in my wardrobe. i have become interested in shopping again, which i haven't been for some time. Thank you, thank you, thank you for giving me the tools to help myself. My daughter is also doing brilliantly (although had little to lose) and we hope one day, maybe next year, to sign up to go on one of Jason's retreats. We are both yoga fans and a week of juicing would be brilliant. We both feel very empowered after reading Jason's books and hope that others will want to share in the success it can bring.

Thanks for the life change ... it continues to be amazing!!
Marianne and Tabitha XXX'

Once again we have someone who simply incorporates a few juices a day into her life and has a balanced evening meal. In her own words: **'Juicing has made steady weight loss EASY,'** something I believe the world is looking for and something you will discover when you start the revolutionary *Juice Yourself Slim* programme.

'Hi Jason

i haven't had a migraine since i started juicing! So i experimented and for a week i didn't juice or exercise (Pilates) and guess what? Yes, my migraine came back with a vengeance! From the time i was a toddler i have suffered from migraines at least once a month, sometimes twice or three times. i have been to several doctors and clinics, done the 'programme', took the pills for 30 years and nothing worked. So thank you Jason and the Juice Master — i am juicing the wheatgrass now with my new juicer. Still doing the Pilates which has helped tremendously with my back injury. And to top it all i have been accepted at the local university to do a design degree. And i'm 60 years young — but where the hell were you for 35 of my years!!!

Thank you again a thousand times.
Penelope P'

I used to suffer from migraines and they aren't a laughing matter. If you have them my heart goes out to you – all you can do is close the world out and pray it goes away soon. This lady is 60 years old and took pills for over 30 years, yet a bit of juicing and some exercise and boom! Problem gone. The juicing and exercise have also helped with a back injury. This isn't the first time I have heard of juicing helping people with migraines.

> ❛ i have lost 23lbs in only four weeks and my asthma has improved so much that i have reduced my medication (i take steroids and have a nebulizer). i wrote to my doctor to make sure it was okay and he's very happy.
>
> Kindest regards
> **Heather** ❜

Most of you will have focused on the massive 23lb weight loss in just four weeks. After all, this book is entitled *Juice Yourself Slim*. However, what I wish to emphasize is that Heather didn't decide to Juice Herself to Lower Asthma Medication – she read the book and wanted to Juice Herself Slim. The improvement in her asthma was a 'side-effect' of the programme.

I used to suffer from severe asthma, to the point where I had steroid tablets and was using my Ventalin inhaler up to 14 times a day, every single day. If I lost my inhaler or misplaced it I would immediately panic, which, not surprisingly, often triggered an attack in itself.

There is no question that diet and environment play a massive role in the development and treatment of this condition. The example above is just one of many I have received over the years from people who are breathing a great deal easier due to a change of diet, increased exercise and, of course, some freshly extracted juice magic. So you may only be doing this to Juice Yourself Slim, but if you suffer from any other condition you may just find that as a side-effect it improves or disappears altogether.

> ❛ i saw a review of your book in one of the health magazines and decided to buy it. i read it from cover to cover and couldn't put it down because i was that keen to start! in six weeks i have lost almost 28lbs, and this has prompted me to get my life into gear.

At 32 i haven't felt or looked better for a long time. Thank you for helping me get my life sorted!

K '

28lbs in six weeks! Now that's the sort of result which should ignite the fire within. Anyone can juice themselves slim and anyone can get these results. All you have to do is read the whole book and then follow the simple *Juice Yourself Slim* programme.

' ... changed my life totally, also saved my life after major surgery. i was in intensive care for two days and couldn't eat. The hospital tried to feed me chips. i got my mother to bring me freshly juiced veg and was home in four days. i had read your book before hospital and knew it worked. The doctors said they had never seen anyone heal so fast. Now i'm just finishing a health and nutrition course, all thanks to the inspiration of Mr Jason Vale.

Thanks pal
Scott '

The doctors said they had 'never seen anyone heal so fast'. Clearly this is anecdotal, but this is far from the first of its kind I have received. I have even had someone suggest they wouldn't be alive today if they hadn't had juice therapy after a large dose of chemotherapy. I am healthily sceptical of such claims, but as I continue to receive similar testimonials, I do believe that healing is improved when the body has the right nutrient elements to work with.

This also illustrates the importance of getting good natural juice bars into hospitals. Our government wastes so much money on various quangos and other money pits so it could easily get a juice bar into all UK hospitals. It's the one place where people's digestive systems are heavily weakened and immune systems compromised. It is also a place where nutrition is looked at as an afterthought. This is despite the fact that 85 per cent of all disease is directly caused by what we put into our mouths, according to the World Health Organization. Juice bars would make money for the hospital and improve the health of the patients, but I guess that's just a little too simple a solution to even consider. On that note, if you have any influence in this area and can help add a genuine Juice Master Natural Juice Bar to some hospitals, please let me know.

'... most recently i purchased 7LBS iN 7 DAYS and decided to give the detox plan a go. i can truly say that i feel better now than in years and have lost a total of 5½ stone. i am looking forward to continuing on my journey through stages two and three, and am eagerly awaiting future book releases from Jason. And yes, i read all of the books all the way through!!

My vital stats, in case you are interested (isn't it amazing how people like to talk about themselves?):

	START	NOW	GOAL
Weight	22st	16½st	16st
Waist	44in	36in	34in
Chest	54in	46in	44in
Feet	Size 12	Size 11	Whatever!

Many thanks and best regards
Adrian '

In case you think he lost 5½ st in seven days, clearly he didn't. The only way that would be possible is by cutting off your legs! This man has been on a two-year journey which started with one of my other books and has continued since. He clearly understands the nature of 'reigniting', and the importance of *continued* reading, learning and inspiration.

As I will repeat constantly throughout the book, life has a habit of coming along and dampening our inspirational flames at times. This is why it is absolutely necessary to do whatever it takes to keep the fire going. We all require some inspirational fuel from time to time, and the right psychological injection can make the difference between being slim for a week and being slim for life.

Although this man had lost 4.5st in just under two years, he needed something to reignite the fire and give him a boost so that he could reach his goal. He got hold of a copy of *7lbs in 7 Days*, read the book, got inspired once again and lost a massive 14lbs in just 7 days! He has a 'Grand Designs' rather than a 'Changing Rooms' approach to his health and fitness goal – something I will explain in depth later – and he is now 5.5st lighter than two years ago.

Super Slimming Success

He's far from the only person to have what I describe as 'super slimming success' using the power of juice and a positive frame of mind. I have had letters from people who have lost over 20st (280lbs), and it's extremely common to receive emails from people who drop three to five stone. The difference that kind of weight loss makes to every aspect of a person's life is almost incalculable.

If you want a small glimpse of what it would feel like, get a rucksack, add 42lbs of weight (21 bags of sugar) and walk around for a day. At the end of the day remove the rucksack and feel the difference. Can you imagine the effect on someone's life of losing three, five or twenty stone? It's often the difference between simply surviving and truly living. It's the difference between being able to get up and play with the kids and a 'can't be bothered' mentality. It's the difference between feeling bloody good about yourself and feeling like crap.

I realize that for many people slimming is the *numero uno* reason for reading this book and doing the programme. But in the same way as understanding the difference significant weight loss makes to someone's life, it's also easy to see how every area of someone's life would be different when they are no longer plagued by migraines, severe asthma, a skin disorder, arthritis, diabetes … and so I could go on. Let's not underestimate the impact this programme will have on all areas of your health, areas which perhaps haven't even manifested themselves yet. Prevention is MUCH easier than cure, and every time you pour some of this 'pure' liquid fuel into your system, you are not only one step closer to the land of the slim, but you are also supplying yourself with perhaps the finest health insurance you will ever invest in.

Fool Proof

I have enough life-changing testimonials to fill an entire book, but for some people these stories won't be enough. It doesn't matter how many genuine letters and emails come in on a daily basis, nor how powerful their stories are – some people need what they consider proof, usually of the 'scientific' kind. Many people in the medical and dietetic professions will see every letter you have just read as purely 'anecdotal' evidence of the effectiveness juices and smoothies have on weight loss and disease, even if it involves freeing themselves of the big C.

Cancer versus Carrots

The cancer-fighting abilities of carrot juice have been well documented, but again no matter how powerful the story I fear it will still be many years before freshly extracted carrot juice is ever prescribed as a prevention or treatment. Dr Bernard Jensen, as far back as the 1930s, illustrated the amazing anti-cancer ability of carrot juice when one of his patients cured himself from what was described as a 'terminal disease' by living on just carrot juice and shots of liquid chlorophyll for one year. He had cancer of the bowel and could hardly eat anything. According to Dr Jensen's reports, doctors had given up on this man. After the year he went back to hospital for a checkup. His hospital report showed that he was **completely free of cancer!**

Another Doctor (Dr H E Kirschner) investigated the story and was so impressed he wrote an article about the effectiveness of fruit and vegetable juices on disease, which he sent to a medical journal. The article was sent back to him explaining, 'the story lacked credibility' and that 'it wasn't up to the medical profession to promote any particular food for the healing of any disease'. I wish to repeat that as it's quite important:

'... it wasn't up to the **medical** profession to promote any particular **food** for the healing of any **disease**'

If it's not up to the medical profession to say what can heal us, whose job is it? The journal also mentioned the story lacked 'credibility'. But the facts are clear: he was diagnosed with terminal bowel cancer. Doctors had sent him home as there was nothing further they could do. He treated his condition with carrots and green juices, and one year later he had no cancer at all. It wasn't as if he made up the fact he had terminal cancer or that it wasn't diagnosed. It was clear he had it and one year later it had vanished. Yes, I agree further studies would be needed before publication of such an article to prove its effectiveness, but that's my point. Instead of looking into it with an open mind and seeing it as a possible breakthrough for the treatment and/or prevention of the big C, it was immediately dismissed as not credible.

This man's case is not an isolated incident either. There have been thousands of cases where carrot juice and liquid chlorophyll have played a positive role in the treatment of cancer and other diseases. This doesn't mean it is a cure for cancer, and it doesn't mean that all medical intervention should stop and carrot juice should take over. That would be foolish. I am simply asking, why isn't the effectiveness of this treatment at least looked at seriously?

Luckily, times are changing. Over the past 10 years in particular there have been many scientific studies carried out with regard to juices and smoothies. These studies appear to back up the health- and life-changing stories of the tens of thousands of emails I have received over the years. Even some members of the dietetic and medical professions are looking into these studies with a degree of seriousness. Genuine testimonials and stories, as we have just seen, are a great way to illustrate the effectiveness of what happens when you add a touch of juicy magic to your daily life. However, for many, what is often even more convincing is when you add ...

3

The Appliance of Juicy Science

When you apply a touch of what is deemed 'scientific evidence' to the health effectiveness of juices and smoothies, more people seem to take notice. And while I believe the best and most reliable 'evidence' for the healing power of fruits and vegetable juices is the hundreds of thousands of *real stories* which have been recorded over the centuries, I am also incredibly open to any genuine scientific study on this subject. Some of the following juice-based scientific evidence is so overwhelming that even the most 'juice sceptic' person out there may well be pursuaded to join the juice therapy revolution.

As this isn't a 'juice study' book, I am providing just a few examples of the theraputic power of fruit and vegetable juices. My hope is that when you see just how effective juices can be when it comes to some quite serious ailments, you will realize just how powerful they will be on what is now the most common disease of all – FAT!

Grape Juice Study Debunks Wine's Health Claims

A study conducted by Dr John D Folts, professor of medicine and director of the Coronary Artery Thrombosis Research and Prevention Laboratory at the University of Wisconsin Medical School, found that purple grape juice is about 66 per cent more effective at treating heart disease than alcohol, but without the harm caused by ethyl alcohol.

Purple grape juice is more effective at treating heart disease than alcohol.

Dr Folts began his studies with a variety of animal species before moving on to human volunteers. Each person in the study had their platelet activity measured half an hour before and after drinking 20–24 ounces (roughly three glasses) of juice. In the studies, purple grape juice in particular reduced platelet activity by more than 40 per cent. This percentage makes it as effective as aspirin therapy for people who are at risk of heart disease. Unlike aspirin, however, grapes have zero adverse side-effects! Also, the flavonoids in purple grape juice remained effective when adrenaline levels in the blood were increased, unlike aspirin. This suggests grape juice may well be more effective than aspirin therapy for people with heart disease. Folts admits more study is required and explains that if someone is taking aspirin therapy they shouldn't just stop and go on grape juice, but he agrees the results look promising.

For years we were told that red wine helps with heart disease. When I wrote *The Easy Way to Stop Drinking* back in 1998, I explained that in no way, shape or form was any positive health effect of wine due to the alcohol. Alcohol is a poison. It is a drug directly and indirectly responsible for over 50,000 deaths in the UK alone, yet at the same time the 'experts' tell us we should have small amounts as it's good for our heart. Why on earth don't they explain that it's not the red wine but the flipping grapes that make the wine? It's the grapes that have the flavonoids, and given grape juice is 66 per cent more effective than the fermented version known as 'wine', doesn't it make sense to juice some fresh grapes if you are concerned about your health rather than knocking back a bottle a wine?

Drinking wine in order to get the antioxidant benefits of grapes is the same as eating Jaffa Cakes to get some vitamin C from the orange flavour inside, or eating a Snickers bar for your daily intake of nuts! For years people said they were drinking Guinness as it was high in iron. However – and this is just a wild stab in the dark – the chances of people actually drinking Guinness simply because they were genuinely worried about their iron count is about as likely as Tom Cruise winning a 'Tallest man in the world' contest. It also seems odd that the people who advocate wine to be 'good for the heart', particularly for men over 40, tend to be male doctors, usually over the age of 40 – umm, funny that.

Apple Juice May Prevent Asthma

The old saying is, 'an apple a day keeps the doctor away', and it appears we can now add 'an apple *juice* a day keeps the doctor away'. Studies have shown that apple juice has many positive health benefits. For example, it has a powerful effect on memory, and can help prevent an often serious condition which is becoming more common by the day – asthma.

Apple juice has a powerful effect on memory and can help prevent asthma.

The National Heart and Lung Institute research, published in the *European Respiratory Journal*, found that children who drank apple juice at least once a day were half as likely to suffer from wheezing as those drinking it less than once a month. Interestingly, the study also concluded that eating fresh apples themselves gave no apparent benefits, illustrating that at times the juice contained within can have even greater health properties than the whole fruit.

There is some evidence that a healthy diet rich in antioxidants and vitamins is good for asthma.

— Dr Mike Thomas, Aberdeen University

Dr Peter Burney, who led the project, said it was possible that 'phyto-chemicals' in apples, such as flavonoids and phenolic acids, were helping to calm the inflammation in the airways, which is a key feature of both wheezing and asthma.

Clearly this doesn't mean if you are taking medicine for asthma you should stop and get a few glasses of apple juice down you. It just once again shows that the natural chemicals which occur in all fruits and vegetables can have a positive effect on all kinds of ailments, including asthma and wheezing. Having been an asthma sufferer myself in the past, I am more than aware of the power of ridding yourself of 'clogging' foods and introducing fresh live foods and juicing into your life. If your system is clogged it's harder to breathe – not rocket science really!

Drinking Juice Slashes Alzheimer's Risk

A recent American-based study found that older people who drank juice three times a week had a **76 per cent** lower chance of developing Alzheimer's disease. Researchers said, 'It was probably due to disease-fighting substances called polyphenols that are naturally found in fruits and vegetables as a possible source of protection.'

> it could offer a relatively **inexpensive** way to fight a disease that ruins **countless** lives and costs the NHS more than cancer, stroke and heart disease put together.
>
> — Dr Milward of the Alzheimer's Research Trust

The study followed nearly 2,000 Japanese-American senior citizens (average age 72) from the Seattle, Washington, area for 10 years. Each participant was free of memory problems or other signs of Alzheimer's at the start of the study. After factoring out other risk factors that may contribute to Alzheimer's disease – such as smoking, years of schooling and exercise habits – the investigators found that people who drank fruit and vegetable juice more than three times a week had a 76 per cent lower risk of developing Alzheimer's disease compared to those who rarely drank juice.

These findings are new and suggest that fruit and vegetable juices may play an important role in delaying the onset of Alzheimer's disease.

— Qi Dai, MD, PhD, Vanderbilt School of Medicine (leader of the study)

This isn't the only study conducted on the effects juicing has on Alzheimer's disease. A team at Glasgow University carried out a study into the benefits of antioxidants. Researchers examined different juices to see what different chemical compounds and level of antioxidants each contained. Results showed that grape, apple and cranberry juices contained the highest amount of beneficial chemicals. Of those, purple grape juice contained the highest and broadest range of polyphenols as well as having the highest antioxidant capacity.

Dietary polyphenols through their antioxidant properties, and possibly other mechanisms, are believed to play a role in protecting against chronic diseases.

— Alan Crozier, Professor of Plant Biochemistry and Human Nutrition, University of Glasgow

Alan Crozier also said, 'Supplementing a healthy diet with a regular intake of a variety of fruit juices such as purple grape juice, grapefruit juice, cloudy apple juice and cranberry juice, will, without major dietary changes, increase the consumer's intake of phenolic antioxidants.'

Scientists have suggested that Alzheimer's disease may be caused by free radicals in the body altering brain cells. As these particular juices are known to supply the body with a good amount of antioxidants, they are perfect for reducing free radical damage, so helping chronic diseases such as Alzheimer's.

Pomegranate Juice Packs a Punch

Helping Treatment of Prostate Cancer

Pomegranate juice, revered by the Ottoman Empire and known in many cultures as the drink of the gods, is proving to be one of the most (if not *the* most) effective treatments for prostate cancer. A study conducted at Jonsson Cancer Centre at UCLA showed that patients with recurrent prostate cancer who drank pomegranate juice after surgery or radiation treatment saw their PSA blood content levels double after about 54 months. Conversely, PSA levels in the same patients prior to drinking the daily 8-ounce doses of pomegranate juice had doubled in just 15 months. The reason why this is so important is that the faster PSA (Prostate Specific Antigen) levels increase in the blood after treatment, *the greater the potential for dying* of prostate cancer.

> We are hoping that **pomegranate** juice offers a novel strategy for **prolonging** the doubling time in men who have been treated for **prostate cancer.**
>
> — Allan Pantuck, MD, associate professor, Department of Urology, David Geffen School of Medicine, UCLA

Pomegranates, like all fruits, are high in antioxidants. Once again, it's these little beauties which have been highlighted in this study. Dr Pantuck went on to say, 'Pomegranate is high in antioxidants, and there is good evidence that inflammation plays an important role in prostate cancer.'

Are you starting to see a pattern here?

Dr Pantuck is the first to explain that pomegranate juice is in no way a cure for prostate cancer as there wasn't one case where PSA levels went to zero, but clearly he does think it is highly effective in prolonging life *after* treatment. My thoughts are if that's the kind of help it can provide after someone has already had this cancer, imagine how powerful this fruit could be in preventing it. Unfortunately, we are still very much a treatment after the fact society, rather than putting the same time and energy into preventing these diseases in the first place.

Pomegranate Juice is Good for the Heart

Studies have also been conducted to look at the effect of pomegranate juice on heart disease. As this juice is packed with antioxidants such as polyphenols, tannins and anthocyanins, it's a powerful weapon in helping repair DNA damage that can lead to a number of serious health conditions, including coronary heart disease. Studies in Israel have shown that daily doses of pomegranate juice prevent the thickening of arteries and slow down cholesterol oxidation by almost half.

FANCY A STIFF DRINK? – POMEGRANATE JUICE HAILED AS 'NATURAL VIAGRA'

Pomegranate juice has also been studied for its effectiveness on erectile dysfunction. In Greece this juice is already a symbol of fertility, and now it appears the chances of finding out have just gone up along with something else. In a US study conducted in 2007, nearly half the men who drank 8fl oz of pomegranate juice with their evening meal said they found it easier to rise to the occasion. Researcher Dr Christopher Forest of the University of California in Los Angeles said, 'Pomegranate juice has great potential in the management of erectile dysfunction.' Pomegranate juice is rich in antioxidants. These increase levels of nitric oxide, which relaxes blood vessel walls. No doubt pharmaceutical companies are now looking at ways to 'isolate' whatever single substance they believe is doing the trick in order to add some chemicals to it, turn it into a drug, get a patent and turn it into a blockbuster. After all, Viagra is one of the most financially successful drugs in history and no 'natural' remedy will ever stand a chance.

Twenty-four Carrot Gold

The high level of betacarotene (pro vitamin A) in carrots is widely believed to be the element that helps in the prevention and treatment of tumours. However, carrots also contain a compound called falcarinol, which protects them from fungal disease. Kirsten Brandt at Newcastle University investigated the effects this natural pesticide had on rats suffering from precancerous tumours. The study concluded that the rats which had raw carrots in their feed were one third less likely to develop full-scale cancerous tumours than those rats which ate a feed free of falcarinol.

When I wrote *Slim 4 Life: Freedom from the Food Trap,* I cited the case of a man who cured his cancer by consuming the fresh juices of carrots, apples, cabbages and leeks. To be clear, he didn't just have a little juice here and there; he went through 75lbs of carrots, 60 apples, six red cabbages and 25lbs of leeks … in a week! Although his cancer was cured completely, the medical profession wasn't impressed and, once again, didn't want to look into it further. Dr Ian Smith, consultant at the Royal Marsden Hospital in London, called the treatment 'scientifically unproven'. While I fully understand why he must come to this conclusion and why it would be unprofessional to say anything else, it frustrates me that calls for a full and thorough study on the back of this are never suggested. Once again, the fact that you cannot patent carrot juice may just play a part here.

In recent years, however, betacarotene has been tested on laboratory rats and mice and has been shown to *prevent* or *reverse* certain types of cancer induced in these lab animals. Again, why are they looking for the 'one aspect' of carrots that help instead of just making organic carrots and their juices compulsory in the treatment of the second most common cause of death in the Western world?

I am not suggesting for one second that there is no place for chemotherapy, radiotherapy and the like. I, unlike some of my 'alternative' colleagues, believe that there is a time and a place for medical help. There are many cases where without chemo, all the juices in the world wouldn't have helped. However, I think juice therapy should be made compulsory after drastic treatment such as chemo. The chemo kills many aspects along with the cancer, and you end up with one incredibly weak and battered system. This is the time when the body is crying out for 'live' nutrients in a form that takes very little energy to digest and eliminate – pure juice is the obvious answer. Of course the ideal scenario is to skip the cancer altogether by giving the body what it needs through raw natural foods and juices *before* anything happens.

Beetroot Juice Reduces Blood Pressure

Drinking 500ml of beetroot juice a day can significantly reduce blood pressure, UK research suggests. In a study conducted at Barts and the London School of Medicine and the Peninsula Medical School, volunteers who drank beetroot juice started to show reductions in blood pressure after just one hour. After just two and a half hours their systolic rate – the pressure with each heartbeat – was around 10 millimetres of mercury (mm Hg) lower than that of participants who had drunk just water. And after just three hours the 'resting' pressure between heartbeats reduced by 8 mm Hg in the juice drinkers. The study's leader, Professor Amrita Ahluwalia from the William Harvey Research Institute at St Bartholomew's Hospital, London, said: 'Drinking beetroot juice, or consuming other nitrate-rich vegetables, might be a simple way to maintain a healthy cardiovascular system and might also be an additional approach that one could take in the modern-day battle against rising blood pressure.'

The key beneficial ingredient appears to be nitrate, which is also found in green, leafy vegetables. But once again I believe it is almost impossible to isolate one specific ingredient found in any fruit or vegetable which is *the* element that makes the difference. Every fruit and vegetable has a naturally balanced blend of vitamins, minerals and co-factors which all combine to furnish the body with the elements required for optimum health. This opinion is echoed by Victoria Taylor of the British Heart Foundation, who said: 'Although we know that eating a diet rich in fruit and vegetables as part of a well balanced diet is beneficial to heart health, we do not know yet whether there are certain fruits or vegetables that are more helpful than others, and so for now people should continue to choose a wide variety in achieving their five a day.'

Oh, and while I'm here, the five a day recommendations are far too light. In Japan the standard recommendations are seventeen portions of fruit and vegetables a day – yes, **SEVENTEEN!** I can't believe the genetic make up of the Japanese is different enough from ours to warrant needing over three times the amount of fruit and vegetable protection as we do. In fact, the government fruit and vegetable recommendations differ from country to country, which I feel means no one has a clue. However, at least all governments are recommending fruit and vegetables, even if the amounts are different.

Beetroot juice is incredibly sweet, yet has a low GI, and when mixed with the juices of apple, celery, cucumber, spinach and a touch of lemon, it tastes delicious.

Cherry Juice to Ease Gout and Muscle Pain

The therapeutic benefits of cherry juice are very well known to those in the 'juice world'. Cherry juice has been used for many years to prevent and help reduce the symptoms of gout and arthritis. Cherries are loaded with flavonoids, which help to reduce high uric acid levels. It is known that high levels of uric acid can lead to the development of gout. In 1950 a study in Texas proved just how effective cherries and cherry juice can be for this condition. Twelve gout sufferers were given the equivalent of 1lb of cherries or cherry juice daily. What they found was that in every case uric acid levels went down to normal and they didn't suffer any more attacks of gouty arthritis. That's *every case!*

Another study, published in the *Journal of Natural Products* in 1999, showed that 20 cherries a day gave similar pain relief to aspirin and other painkillers as they inhibited compounds that caused inflammation in the joints.

It's not just cherries that help with this condition. Pomegranate, blueberries, hawthorn and any dark-red berries contain these beneficial flavonoids.

No Pain — Plenty of Gain

If you are a gym bunny (and if you're not I hope this book inspires you to start moving your body on a regular basis) you may be interested to know that cherry juice has also been studied for its effectiveness on exercised-induced pain and damage. Dr Norman Walker (the late great juicing pioneer) illustrated how effective a combination of celery, cucumber and apple juice can be on helping to reduce lactic acid buildup after working out. However, it appears cherry (or any dark berry) juice is even more effective.

Cherry juice has been shown to help reduce muscle pain after exercise.

Scientists at the University of Vermont found that recovery time was a great deal faster and muscle pain was reduced with the help of a little pre-exercise cherry and apple juice. The study also illustrated that muscle strength showed signs of improvement after only 96 hours. Whether it was the apple juice combined with the cherry juice, the flavonoids, the natural balance of sodium and potassium or whatever, one thing is getting clearer and clearer – juice works. Often people don't know why and how it works, but seemingly no matter what the condition, this super-charged liquid works, even in areas where medicine has failed.

Juice for Breakfast Builds Bones in Rats

This study may sound a little more science fiction than science fact, but as osteoporosis affects millions of people worldwide, it may be worth taking note. Researchers in Texas have discovered that a little citrus juice can go a long way to strengthening bones. They found that orange and grapefruit juice regularly given to lab rats *prevented* osteoporosis, a condition which has long been considered an unavoidable aging disease in which bones become more likely to break.

A reduction in bone density is often caused when there is an increase in oxidants. Clearly, both grapefruit juice and orange juice increased antioxidants in the rats' systems, which is probably one of the reasons behind the success of the experiment. However, as there are over 400 known compounds in citrus it would be hard to know which specific element made the difference. But why look for 'the' element? Why not just know that, for whatever reason, it works. So instead of trying to find the 'magic' within to create a drug pill, why don't we just drink more juice? Just a thought!

It's not the first time citrus has been cited as a 'major breakthrough' for a particular disease. A study has also shown how oranges and grapefruit are:

Powerful in the Fight against Breast Cancer and High Cholesterol

Researchers from the Centre for Human Nutrition at the University of Western Ontario, Canada, have found a link between orange and grapefruit juice and the treatment of breast cancer and high LDL (bad) cholesterol. Dr Kenneth Carroll, director of the centre, said, 'The implications are potentially enormous because a powerful weapon against breast cancer and high cholesterol may be as close as your kitchen.' However, there really isn't anything new here. Hippocrates – known as 'the father of medicine' – famously said, 'Let food be thy medicine.' And the kind of food he was talking about was the high-liquid, raw, 'live' fuel provided by nature.

'Mice that received orange juice or grapefruit juice in place of drinking water had 50 per cent fewer tumours and metastases,' said Najla Guthrie, lead researcher on the centre's cancer study. 'The study groups receiving flavonoids also had a reduction in tumours, but not to the extent of the groups receiving juices. This leads us to believe that in the juice study groups, the flavonoids were working with other components in the juices to reduce the tumours.'

The last point made is critical. Note that the flavonoids given by themselves had a significantly *lower* impact in reducing tumours. The researchers believe that the results were so much better in the juice study groups due to the flavonoids working with other components in the juices to reduce the tumours. But is it me or **ISN'T IT BLOODY OBVIOUS?!** As I mentioned not long ago, it seems mad when scientists try to find 'the' component within the juice, fruit or veg which is working the magic. Isn't it clear that there are possibly millions of components all working together to bring life and fight disease?

I am talking here about something that isn't tangible, which can never be truly scientific – an X factor if you will. An X factor contained within the life-giving liquid fuel which no person on earth – no matter what title they have or how many letters after their name – will ever be able to fully replicate. How else can you explain not only the results of many scientific studies conducted on juice but, more importantly, the thousands of letters and astounding emails which show, time and time again, this unique and powerful X factor in action?

Super Juice Me!

For research for this book, 10 volunteers went on an *exclusive* diet of fresh juices and smoothies for 30 days. The idea was to see what would happen to them on a mental and physical level. The research came about as a direct result of the successes people had on the seven-day juice-only programme. It was also inspired by Morgan Spurlock's groundbreaking documentary *Super Size Me*.

In his film, Spurlock lived on nothing but McDonald's for 30 days and documented what happened. He had a range of health tests before, during and after the fast food experiment. Even before the end of the research doctors warned him not to continue as part of his liver had literally turned to mush and he was in danger of causing permanent damage to himself. The documentary illustrated the potential harm that can happen in a very short space of time when you clog your system with junk and lack essential nutrients. The documentary had its flaws, but overall the message was clear.

I wanted to know what would happen if instead of super-sizing someone and making them dangerously ill, you 'super-juiced' them and made them super healthy and super slim. I was extremely curious. I thought, if people are losing 7–14lbs in just one week on a juice and smoothie exclusive 'diet', what kind of change would be seen if they continued on nothing but juice for 10, 20 or even 30 days? I wondered what would happen not only in terms of super weight loss, but also with every aspect of mental and physical wellbeing. Here is a letter I have just received from one of the volunteers:

‘ Hiya

i have to say i feel amazing. So, so happy and refreshed.

My poor skin has cleared up, my asthma has improved (i can actually go upstairs without almost dying at the top), my hair is shiny and healthy looking, and i've not even finished yet!

The main change to my life has been that my periods have started again. When i was 18 i was diagnosed with PCOS (polycystic ovarian syndrome). i was told there was a good chance i would have trouble conceiving when i came to want children. i have since read more about it and realize the diagnosis they gave me was a bit too gloomy, but i've still lived with the fact that i may never have children.

i also know that part of the condition is weight gain, and that weight is normally harder to lose. But i think i've used this as an excuse for far too long. i've proved with the help of this programme that it's not that hard to lose weight and be healthy. i've resisted the temptation to weigh myself so far, but i have measured myself and the results look really, really promising.

in the 10 years since my diagnosis i've only had around 10 periods, and only when i've been given something to bring them on. My weight has slowly crept on and on until i knew that i was building something around me to prevent me from getting close to partners. That way the issue of kids would never come up.

Now i feel like i've been given my future back! My first natural period in 10 years has to be a good sign. Maybe i can be a healthy weight where the fact that i have PCOS doesn't hold me back from having a family of my own.

i'm so excited about the future and what it holds for me. i will let you know the final results of my trial when i get them. Please let me know if you need anything else.

Kind regards
Tasha X

Once again, you will have most in the dietetic and medical world dismissing the above as 'purely anecdotal' and 'non-scientific', but sometimes I think we simply have to accept that even if we have studied a particular subject for years, we may not necessarily know all the answers. I certainly don't and I never pretend to either.

Science can't explain how this woman got her first natural period for 10 years, and I guess neither can anyone in the medical or alternative field. All we know is that when we stop putting in rubbish and supply the body with plenty of nutritious, high-water-content plant foods and drinks instead, the body heals. Why? Who knows? Does it matter as long as people get well?

This was far from the only amazing result from the Super Juice Me! trial programme. Those who completed the programme to the letter (and as you can imagine it wasn't everyone, as living on *nothing* but juice for 30 days has its challenges!) lost anything from 14lbs to as much as 28lbs (that's 2 stone or 12 kilos!). They also lost many inches from the areas that matter, and many aspects of their health improved immeasurably. The 'before' and 'after' stats (blood pressure, cholesterol, BMI, sugar levels and so on) show some good improvements. Those looking from a scientific perspective will no doubt find some of the results impressive, and others okay and inconclusive. However, what these stats don't show are stories like Tasha's, above. They don't show how someone feels, or the health problems that were eliminated. Nor do they show changes to energy levels and their general outlook on life. The real results are almost intangible and can only be truly appreciated when you hear directly from the juicer's mouth – so to speak.

‘Hi Jason

Just to update you on the fantastic results from the 30-day trial. Well, we finished juicing last Thursday and not only have we lost about 18lbs EACH but we feel absolutely fantastic. My blood pressure has come down slightly, i did not have a migraine in the 30 days (unheard of for me), my mood swings have been non-existent (my doctor confirmed before i began that i have actually started the menopause ... oh joy), my stomach is lovely and flat and two people have commented on my radiant complexion!!!!! it has been so well worth doing and, to be honest, i am really missing the discipline of juicing. We are now having a juice in the morning for breakfast, salad for lunch and fish and vegetables/salad or soup in the evening. We are currently experimenting with healthy foods and totally enjoying it.

Also, for John it has stopped his reflux, he looks and feels years younger and has stopped snoring!! Thank you for giving us the opportunity to take part. it has made us stop and re-evaluate our life, and i must say we definitely do now have an attitude of gratitude.

Annette X’

Where do we start? Their stats on paper showed me their weight loss and improvements in blood pressure, fat percentages and BMI (body mass index). However, I didn't see the real results until I received the above email. Previously I didn't know Annette's mood swings had become non-existent – not gone down a little – **NON-EXISTENT!** I also didn't know about the migraines, the flat stomach, the radiant complexion, the no snoring. And I didn't know from the stats alone that they are 'feeling absolutely fantastic'. This is what science often can't show and what so often simply gets dismissed as 'purely anecdotal' and 'an isolated case'. Yet it's where I feel the real juice lies.

This isn't to dismiss the scientific studies illustrated earlier and throughout this chapter as they all add weight to the juicy argument. Some are extremely useful and help to illustrate the possibilities of juice therapy as a recognized and serious treatment in years to come. I just feel hearing the stories from real people illustrates much more than looking at the effect betacarotene has on a rat.

> **'Dear Jason**
>
> i absolutely love your books. You may be interested to know that i gave one to a friend who had been diagnosed with bladder cancer. He totally switched to juicing, and when his bladder was recently checked under anaesthetic at the hospital in Aberdeen, he was told that there are now no cancer cells at all.
>
> The doctors asked what my friend was doing and he told them he was juicing broccoli, cauliflower, cabbage and so on, which have been found by Harvard Medical School to kill bladder cancer cells. The doctors were amazed at how healthy my friend's bladder now looks. He puts it all down to my giving him your book to read, which went into all the amazing nutrients in fruit and vegetables. **'**

My mother's husband died of bladder cancer and I know at first hand that it's not a pretty disease. The above email is quite astonishing. Again, I am not saying that if you have bladder cancer you will cure it with juicing, but I am saying it is clear that juicing needs to be looked at seriously, especially when you get miracle results like this. This man juiced broccoli, cauliflower and cabbage and now he has a healthy bladder. A bladder where cancer cells once were.

This isn't 'scientific' as such, but I feel it's incredibly impressive by any standards and even more reason why natural juice therapy should be looked at as an alternative to drug treatment and/or used in combination with it. I am doing all I can to get natural juice therapy recognized as a legitimate treatment of disease, as well as a preventive therapy. To do this I have teamed up with Dr E Taylor and a top UK university. As I write, the course has just been accepted by the CMA (Complementary Medical Association). If you are interested in helping people via the power of natural juice therapy, you can apply to join our ever-expanding team of Juice Master Natural Juice Therapists around the world (*see page 287*).

What is Science Anyway?

Well, according to the *Oxford English Dictionary*, the definition is, 'the intellectual and practical activity encompassing the systematic study of the structure and behaviour of the physical and natural world through observation and experiment'. So that's cleared that up then!

The problem is we tend to be so accepting of science – whatever our understanding of it – that we rarely, if ever, question it over common sense. We also rarely understand that what is often deemed 'scientific fact' is no more than scientific opinion or theory. After all, 'the world is flat' was once deemed scientific fact, as was the 'fact' that an atom could never be split. Scientific 'fact' is based on a conclusion from evidence presented at the time.

As humans we tend to be obsessed with what we consider to be our own 'intelligent breakthroughs' in the world of treatments or preventative therapies. So much so that we can be blind to what can only be described as the 'flipping obvious'. It is, after all, obvious that there are many different components contained within the liquid of nature's foods, which all combine in a unique way to help with the treatment and prevention of disease. It is also obvious that you cannot expect to isolate just one element within the fruit or vegetable juice, make a synthetic version of it and get the same results as the 'live' liquid. Clearly we need scientific study. All I am saying is we need a touch of common sense too.

Nature has provided us with the finest medicine and fuel in the form of high-water-content 'live' foods. I don't know why this life-giving liquid is so effective in the treatment and prevention of seemingly every disease known to man – it just is. I also don't fully understand why it's so highly effective with permanent *healthy* weight loss – I just know it is! Sometimes the most intelligent thing to do is *not* get bogged down with the whys and wherefores and just have some trust and faith. If you end up with much better health and a super-slim body after this programme, do you really care why it worked?

Nature has provided us with the finest medicine and fuel in the form of 'live' foods.

One Big Fat Global Problem

Fat is now a global issue. There are more overweight people in the Western world than ever before, and our junkie food and Nintendo generation is spilling over to the East at a rapid rate. We have more obese children than ever and we know the situation in the US. And while we have all been growing fatter and sicker, more anti-fat drug pills have come on to the market than at any other time in history. Clearly they are having zero effect on the problem, yet more and more keep being scientifically tested, each one with a clean bill of health and medically 'proven to help'.

It's not that governments aren't taking the obesity issue seriously. As I write, the UK government has just announced that it wants to increase the ban on advertising junk food on television, while at the same time warning, 'Obesity is as serious as climate change.' What they aren't doing is looking at things like juice therapy as seriously as drug therapy. When I say *as seriously*, I mean they aren't looking at it at all. Indeed, they often claim it's dangerous – yes, fruit and vegetable juice 'dangerous'. You really can't make this stuff up!

Big Food — Big Pockets

On top of this there are large moves to 'ban' any alternative treatment which hasn't been 'scientifically' tested. In fact, food companies will soon no longer be able to claim that their products are 'good for your heart', 'help to lower cholesterol' or are one of the growing list of 'super-foods' unless they have scientific backing. This is the result of a new European Nutrition and Health Claims Regulation designed to 'help protect consumers from misleading claims'. On the surface this is a very good thing, but notice it states '*unless* they have scientific backing'. This means the **BiG FOOD** companies – the ones with the **BiG MONEY** – can easily pay for any independent scientific study to be done on their food or drink. These studies are usually a long way from genuine scientific evidence and at times, far from independent.

This means that we will see more and more adverts from **BiG FOOD** companies making claims such as 'helps to lower cholesterol' and 'can help to maintain a healthy heart', while the genuine health benefits of many *pure* and natural foods and drinks will never be allowed to be displayed.

For example as I write this there is a very expensive advertising campaign for 'Flora pro.activ'. The heading of the advert reads in big bold letters:

NO FOOD LOWERS CHOLESTEROL MORE

It then has the subheading, 'Lots of foods can help lower cholesterol, but no food lowers cholesterol more than Flora pro.activ …' Now, I am not suggesting that Flora has done anything wrong with advertising its product in this way, but surely in order for this statement to be factually correct every single food on earth would have to be tested for its cholesterol-lowering properties. There is no way this was done. They also have 'Flora – Love Your Heart' on the magazine ad. They no doubt aren't saying anything wrong and are allowed to write this about their product, due to the strong belief in and scientifically-backed research into the Diet-Heart Hypothesis (aka The Cholesterol Hypothesis). This hypothesis states that high LDL (Low Density Lipoproteins, also known as 'bad cholesterol') is the cause of heart disease and if you lower LDL cholesterol you won't get a heart attack or stroke, and is taken as read by most in the medical profession. However, according to some doctors, this could not be completely accurate. Dr Malcolm Kendrick, author of the must-read *The Great Cholesterol Con*, has strong evidence which shows heart disease isn't caused by raised cholesterol at all, but rather a combination of many other contributing factors including obesity, smoking and stress. If this somewhat unorthodox view is correct, then it will not be welcome news to the **BiG DRUGS** who are currently raking in billions from the 'print money' pills known as statins. At the time of writing two million people in the UK are taking 'cholesterol lowering' drugs and I can guarantee that by the time you read this, due to 'safe cholesterol levels' being lowered all the time, it will be much, much, **MUCH** higher. After all, lower the safe cholesterol level by even a small fraction, from say 5 to 4, and you have a situation where millions more are all of a sudden in 'danger' and must be treated immediately.

... I digress slightly ... where were we? Oh yes ... There was, unbelievably, even a suggestion that statins should be added to our drinking water. What happened to the law which states they cannot medicate without our express permission? It seems as if it might be about to go out of the window ... oh sorry, I forgot, they've already added fluoride to our drinking water ...

I am all for regulation and protection against 'snake oil' potions, and stopping unscrupulous individuals from taking advantage of the public, especially when it comes to their health. At the same time, however, our right to know exactly what natural remedies have genuinely helped needs to be upheld. I have already illustrated how nuts it is that we have a ruling stating that *only* a drug can 'prevent, treat or cure disease', despite the fact fruits and vegetables have been proven beyond any reasonable doubt to do all three things to various degrees. So it should come as no surprise that the bigger the SICK business gets, the more restrictions will be put on any 'alternative' to drug therapy. It is also ironic that this new ruling has come in before a crackdown has occurred on the massive corruption in the 'scientifically tested' drug world.

There was even a call recently to prevent goji berries from being sold in the UK because there was no proof they weren't harmful and they hadn't been fully tested. But 'fully tested' on whom? These magnificent red berries have been around probably since the dawn of time, and each 100 grams contains:

- 112mg calcium (10 per cent of Recommended Daily Allowance, RDA)
- 1132mg potassium (24 per cent RDA)
- 9mg iron (100 per cent RDA)
- 2mg zinc (18 per cent RDA)
- 50mcg selenium (91 per cent RDA)
- 1.3mg riboflavin (100 per cent RDA)
- 29mg vitamin C (32 per cent RDA)
- 7mg betacarotene
- 25–200mg zeaxanthin
- 31g polysaccharides

They also stimulate the release of remunerative human growth hormones by the pituitary gland and have been used for centuries for strength building, helping to regulate blood sugar and improve sleep and vision. Oh, and they have never caused any AGRs (adverse goji reactions)! I don't think there has been any 'scientific evidence' to show that oranges aren't harmful – or pears, pineapple or grapefruit for that matter. You can't imagine someone trying to ban the sale of fruit and veg because there was no evidence it doesn't do harm, but that's exactly what is happening with things like goji berries. After all, they're only bloody berries!

Around eight million people take 1g of vitamin C supplement every day. However, this practice will come to an end by the close of 2009, not because the supplements have been found to be harmful, but because Brussels says so! It's not just vitamin C up for a ban: almost 5,000 'alternative' products used by millions of people, with the sole objective of trying to help themselves on the health front, will be banned. Yes, vitamins and minerals banned – has the world gone bonkers? No, I fear it has just got even greedier. Let's face facts, **BIG PHAR-MACIES** don't want anyone stepping on their turf, and the banning of alternative remedies has always been on the cards because of their potential to interfere with the profits of some of the most influential companies on earth. Sceptical of such claims? Think I'm just paranoid and that government and drug companies are there to look out solely for our best interest and not theirs? Well, let's look at a little case history which may at least enable you to keep an open mind and not simply buy into what you hear, even if it comes as official advice from government.

On 4 July 1997, not long after Tony Blair came to power, Jeff Rooker, the minister of state at the Ministry of Agriculture, Fisheries and Food (MAFF) issued a press release. On the advice of the Committee on Toxicity (CoT), Mr Rooker planned, on health grounds, to introduce drastic restrictions on the sale of products containing ... wait for it ... vitamin B6. No, I'm not joking. The Labour government wanted to prevent thousands of health shops selling dietary supplements containing vitamin B6 in what they considered to be high doses, allowing them to sell in quantities of just 10mg. Anything higher would only have been available from pharmacies and would have needed a license from the Medicines Control Agency (MCA). Anything above 50mg would even have required a doctor's prescription! It's worth knowing that an estimated three million people in the UK use vitamin B6 on a regular basis, meaning it is an incredibly profitable business. When B6 is deficient it can lead to insomnia, loss of libido, depression and a host of other disorders. The new ruling would have inevitably instantly handed over the very profitable B6 market to the pharmaceutical industry, the only ones who could have afforded the huge sums of money required to get each B6 product licensed, under EC law, by the MCA. The MCA, it is worth noting, relies on the pharmaceutical companies for its income.

An overwhelming campaign against the proposed restrictions involving Rooker's peers, the public and genuine science meant he had no alternative but to back down and not go ahead with the ban ... *for now*. It is worth knowing that despite the fact that there has not been a single scientifically-proven case of toxicity recorded from B6 at doses of 500mg or below, in 2007 the Food Standards Agency was advising against taking more than 10mg of vitamin B6 supplements a day. But why? It doesn't make any sense at all.

I am more than aware of the drive to seemingly prevent any alternative natural food remedy from being sold. On my own range of pure supplements I can't use certain terms, such as what vitamins and minerals they contain (no, I'm not making it up!). My range of Juice Boosters only came about because there are many amazing fruits and vegetables which either you can't get fresh in the UK or can't be juiced or blended. They are picked at their ripest and dried at very low temperatures to preserve the enzyme activity. Spirulina, for example, is a blue green algae that has 10 times more calcium than milk, 58 times more iron than spinach and is a complete protein. But can I put that on the label? Not a chance! I developed my Clear Skin Booster from my own 20 years of research battling with psoriasis. Not one medical treatment cures this condition and they ALL have adverse side-effects, some horrific. They have also all been 'scientifically tested' and can all state, 'helps in the treatment of psoraisis'. Despite the fact all of the ingredients contained within my powder have been reported as having a positive effect on skin conditions – and despite the fact I only produced it to help myself due to the inefficiency in this area by the medical profession – I still cannot make any claim with relation to skin conditions. I also wouldn't be surprised if I soon had to rename it altogether, till in the end it just says, 'harmless powder you can add to a juice'!

Doesn't it seem crackers for the authorities to try and ban natural foods such as goji berries and yet products like Sunny Delight were, hey, okay from the start? A product which clearly deceived many parents into thinking they were getting natural orange juice, when in fact the drink was about as far from pure orange juce as you can get. Trans-fats are still readily available in our foods, and E numbers – known to cause hyperactivity and God knows what else – are also loaded in many foods and, ironically, medicines. The blockbuster drug world has more influence than we often realize and it wouldn't surprise me if we soon had new legislation which prevents the sale of any 'alternative' health product, no matter how safe.

> **Trans-fats are still readily available in our foods, and E numbers — known to cause hyperactivity and God knows what else — are also loaded in many foods and, ironically, medicines.**

Living in an 'Obesogenic' Society

The largest ever UK study into obesity, backed by the government and compiled by 250 experts, said excess weight was now the norm in our 'obesogenic' society. No you haven't misread: 'obesogenic' is the new fat word on the block, and by the time you read this it may be widespread. Obesogenic comes from the words 'obese' and 'genic' and describes a society of high-fat food, hours of television watching and lack of physical movement. Every year, overweight and obesity cost the UK nearly £7 billion in treatment and state benefits and in indirect costs such as loss of earnings and reduced productivity. That's **SEVEN BILLION POUNDS,** a figure which is hard to get your head around. The report showed the situation is getting worse every year, and unless something is done *now* we will have a health crisis which will bring the NHS to its knees (although it's nearly there already – have you tried to get treatment recently?). It's not like we are talking about cancer here, where we genuinely don't have a cure as such. We are talking about excess fat, or obesity, a disease for which everyone – regardless of any nutritional study – can blatantly see what the cure is. I mean, it's not rocket science, is it?

Obesogenic comes from the words 'obese' and 'genic' and describes a society of high-fat food, hours of television watching and lack of physical movement.

Starting a 'Leptogenic' Movement

What we are aiming for is a 'leptogenic society', not an obesogenic one. Leptogenic comes from the Greek *leptos* – thin/fine or delicate – and means *leading to weight loss*. It is the direct opposite of obesogenic. In order for us to get a society which is 'leading to weight loss', we need to take our *internal* environment just as seriously as the external one. Not to do so can only be described as a little …

4

Environ Mental!

Pollution and the environment are political hot potatoes at the moment and everyone has an opinion on the subject. The jury is still out on whether we are to blame for global warming and what, if anything, we can do to prevent it. It's also another area where scientists are disagreeing vehemently, which makes it hard for the layperson to know who to listen to. After all, if science is set in stone, why is there such difference of opinion on the same subject? Not that you would know there is a difference of opinion in the science world on this subject as we are – as is so often the case – bombarded with just one side of the argument. Even the 'impartial' BBC has a one-sided opinion on global warming.

If I were sceptical and perhaps cynical, I might think the 'environment' was the perfect fear-based subject that all good governments could use to add more tax to everything we do in the name of 'saving the world'. After all, fear is a great emotional driver, and if you also make it 'cool' to be seen green whilst at the same time making anyone with an opposing view feel like scum, you are on to one hell of a financial winner in the name of 'caring'. However, I would only say such things if I were a conspiracy theorist, but I am not, so I won't.

The Inconvenient Truth

The inconvenient truth is that the man-made global warming theory is just that, a theory. It's simply a hypothesis and despite what virtually everyone reports, it is **NOT** a fact at all. However, if, unlike myself, you do believe that man is the cause of global warming – and its not simply a normal part of this living, breathing entity known as earth – there is an extremely simple way we can all help. What's wonderful is that by adopting this extremely easy measure not only will you be able to sleep soundly and smugly knowing you are 'doing your bit', you be helping in so many other areas too (more about that at the end of this chapter).

Our internal Environment

When it comes to our internal environment the answers are just a little clearer. When I say a little clearer, I mean bloody obvious. You don't need a science degree to realize if we stop polluting and essentially poisoning our systems with an excessive amount of junk and start feeding it the correct nutrients – *everything* will get better. This isn't up for debate; it's as clear as it gets.

Louis Pasteur was one of the first to point to a 'one disease' hypothesis – the theory that although we may have several 'symptoms' of disease, they are all in fact a direct result of just one disease. This one disease can be caused by a chemical deficiency as well as levels of toxicity in the body. The chemical deficiency is simply caused by years of nutritional neglect and can easily be rectified with organic juicing. When a person comes up 'chemically short', body tissues start to malfunction and the resulting symptoms are then named according to how they manifest themselves and treated as 'disease'. Dr Bernard Jensen, author of *Juicing Therapy: Nature's Way to Better Health and a Longer Life*, sums it up beautifully:

Sixteen thousand symptoms and symptom combinations have been recorded for the different ailments, disturbances and diseases ... **every** single one of these symptoms can be helped with nutritional means, especially through the use of **fresh fruit** and **vegetable juices.**

That's **SiXTEEN THOUSAND DiFFERENT SYMPTOMS,** including everything from skin rashes to bowel problems. Sixteen thousand different names for what is, when looked at its simplest and with a dash of common sense, essentially the same disease. Yes, we may have different names for all these symptoms and symptom combinations, but don't they all stem from a constant and steady stream of inner environment pollution?

Inner pollution is caused by external pollution from city living, passive smoking and so on, as well as by stress and negative thinking. The 'foods' and 'drinks' we consume can also clog our systems, slowly but surely, on a *daily* basis. It is only due to the body's incredible natural survival mechanism that we don't all suffer earlier. In fact, it is amazing just how much inner pollution the body can put up with and still survive without any *obvious* signs of disease. I smoked three packets of cigarettes a day, drank alcohol like it was going out of fashion and shovelled junk into my body on a daily basis. Yet, amazingly, I am still here. I am not entirely sure I would still be here if I hadn't started to drink nature's finest fuel on a regular basis. I had many symptoms of disease – not quite sixteen thousand – but it is interesting to read from Dr Jensen that all of the sixteen thousand symptoms 'can be helped by nutritional means, *especially* through the use of fruit and vegetable juices'. This is why when people start to juice themselves slim, many other aspects of their general wellbeing improve, often dramatically. My asthma went, my skin got better, I lost weight and my energy increased.

When people start to juice themselves slim, many other aspects of their general wellbeing improve, often dramatically.

One Big Fat Disease

Isn't it blooming obvious that it's this *inner pollution* which is the real cause of arthritis, eczema, heart disease, cancer, migraines, IBS and most of modern day disease, including **FAT?** Doesn't it seem strange that wild animals suffer a minute fraction, if any, of the disease of humans? Cancer is almost unknown in the wild, heart disease is hardly threatening your average wild giraffe or rhino and you won't see many penguins unable to move properly due to a terrible arthritic condition they have. You also won't see many, if any, obese wild animals. I agree something like an elephant may look overweight, and some gorillas may have a touch of the 'Buddha in a bath', but that's just their build. All elephants and gorillas are the same shape – unlike humans. It is also odd, don't you think, that the only animals who suffer the exact same diseases as ourselves are the domesticated ones or ones in captivity – in other words the ones *we* feed! Your average chimpanzee, our closest living relative, lives on average for 180 years – yes, 180 years. They also die with ALL of their teeth still very much firmly in their mouth. No dentist – no doctor – no NHS!

So what's the difference, you may ask? Well, put simply, raw 'live' organic *water-rich* foods. In the wild, every single animal consumes its food raw and organic. All raw food has 'life energy'. You won't find a cooker in the wild, and all plant-eating animals are getting a regular supply of natural organic nutrient-rich water every time they eat. This is the very essence of the X factor which juice therapy provides. It is the very reason why many 'miracles' occur when you simply replace a few meals a week with some pure fruit and, more importantly, *green* vegetable-based juices and smoothies.

People often worry that they will want to eat their own arm off when replacing a meal with a smoothie. However, they usually find they are completely satiated. Most people are overfed and undernourished. When they begin to top up their chemical deficiency with natural, chemically rich liquid fuel and feed their body on a cellular level, they become genuinely fed using far fewer calories. This all adds up to eating *less*, being nourished *more* and getting a stronger immune system, whilst helping any aliments you currently have (even the ones that haven't fully manifested themselves yet). The more we cook our food, the more we denature it and the more it turns into something potentially harmful.

'Cooked Food is Linked to Cancer in Women'

This headline appeared on the front page of a UK national newspaper in 2007. This was on the back of a Dutch study which found that levels of the chemical acrylamide – which is produced when certain foods are fried, roasted or grilled – are heavily linked to some cancers, especially ovarian and womb cancer.

Although the FSA (Food Standards Agency) welcomed the report saying, 'This new study supports our current advice and policy, which already assumes that acrylamide has the potential to be a human carcinogen,' they also said, 'Since acrylamide forms naturally in a wide variety of cooked food it is not possible to have a healthy balanced diet that avoids it.' This statement is, of course, absolute nonsense. It's like saying wild animals cannot possibly have a healthy balanced diet unless they cook some of their food. Notice they say, 'acrylamide forms naturally in a wide variety of cooked food'. How can it occur naturally? You have to cook the food to make it occur. Acrylamide *only* occurs in cooked food. Cooked food is only eaten by humans and the animals we feed. And virtually every major disease occurs only in humans and the animals we feed. In the wild, where animals consume *only* raw food, disease is virtually unknown and harmful chemicals like acrylamide don't exist.

Personally, I think the study, like many, is flawed for many reasons. I also think that our systems have evolved enough to eat some cooked food and still thrive. I should imagine that you would have to consume a huge amount of acrylamide in order for it to cause cancer. However, the study suggested that if you were to eat just one packet of crisps or a bag of chips you could be in danger. I feel we really should give the body much more credit than that.

Having said that, it is virtual suicide to eat a diet of virtually nothing but cooked and processed foods. Raw food protects, heals and nourishes. A well-protected body can easily deal with quite a large degree of cooked and processed food, but without a daily dose of 'live' liquid nutrition, the body's defences are heavily compromised and we come up chemically short. Synthetic chemical drugs and vitamin and mineral tablets *cannot fill this void*. It can only be filled with the X factor stuff contained within raw organic plants designed for human consumption.

The average 'live' apple today has only a fifth of the nutrition contained in apples 50 years ago. This is because we have over-farmed and bastardized our soil so much in the name of profit. However, once you process that apple by shoving it in a can swimming in sugary water, it is reported that you would need to eat 100 times more to get the same nutritional value as found in the apple. That's **ONE HUNDRED TIMES!** This is why in today's corporate food world of profit at any cost, it is extremely easy to come up chemically short. And, as I will repeat throughout this book, when you are chemically and nutritionally short, you will always be hungrier than you should be, eat more and thus gain weight. This extra hunger is exactly what the mass-market food world wants. More hunger equals more money!

Feeding Off Your Hunger

I mentioned earlier that the **BiG FOOD** manipulators are legally obliged to increase their profits. The *only* way they can do this is to cut many corners with the food they produce and/or induce more hunger. I wrote about this in *Slim 4 Life: Freedom from the Food Trap* and I was the first person to start exposing what I referred to as the 'drug food' companies. I thought at the time that it was simply the white refined sugar causing all the 'false hungers'. After further investigation over the years, however, I now realize that many 'food' companies add chemicals with the sole purpose of making you hungrier. The hungrier you get, the fatter you become and the more money they get.

Foods containing these chemicals that create false hunger are often short on chemicals which the body actually needs. So you have a double whammy: your body calls for more food on a cellular level as it is genuinely being starved, *plus* it is loaded with chemicals that have been designed to cause even more hunger. So, to put it simply, you are screwed! The *only* way to solve this problem is to chemically enrich your body with the finest organic nutrient-packed juices, to eat excellent quality foods the vast majority of the time and to move your body on a regular basis.

I will cover food, what to look out for on labels and so on a little later, but please, please, please never *ever* underestimate what corporate food and drink companies will do in the name of profit. It's not your health that is of concern; it's the health of their bank accounts and making sure they are keeping their shareholders happy campers. Oh, and please don't think for one second that the FSA (Food Standards Agency) will protect you either. The corporate mass-market food world has a degree of corruption on *every* level. The agency has allowed things into our food like hydrogenated oil, aspartame (known as NutraSweet), monosodium glutamate and more E's than an 80s rave, even though stacks of research shows how potentially harmful and addictive they can be. Perhaps, then, we shouldn't fully trust them to keep our food truly safe and nutritionally rich. The agency has had complaint after complaint about certain 'foods' and 'drinks', yet nothing, seemingly, is ever done. I am not saying they are corrupt – I even know people who work on their behalf and are more than credible – I am just asking the question based on the fact that known harmful chemicals are in perfectly legal food and drinks that are still being sold today.

Let's not forget that cocaine was allowed in Coke years ago, a substance added *only* for its addictive qualities. Now, of course, it's the caffeine and sugar doing the trick. Also, let's not forget that cigarettes were once hailed as a health product – yes, cigarettes good for your health. You really can't make this stuff up! Trust is such a fragile thing and we should be able to trust the people whom *we* pay to protect us from harm to do their job efficiently with no conflict of interests of any kind.

Unfortunately, the world is far, far more corrupt than we will ever really know and **BiG FOOD** has big pockets. There is a great deal of money in making people fatter and hungrier whilst fooling them into believing they are being looked after. As early as the 1950s the tobacco companies knew how harmful and addictive their products were, yet it took many, many years before the truth came out. Even today, some of the big cigarette companies are still refusing to admit the truth, despite the overwhelming evidence.

There is no question that exactly the same is happening with certain aspects of the 'food' and 'soft drink' industry. I can guarantee that one day it will come out how some **BiG FOOD** companies added certain chemicals to our food to increase hunger and profits in exactly the same way cigarette companies added *more* nicotine simply to make them more addictive. If in 1950 I had suggested cigarette companies were doing this and they knew how harmful their products were, I would be in court faster than you can say 'Marlborough Lights'. Today, to suggest any food company would even contemplate such a thing seems outrageous, but remember where you heard it first.

I digress again … back with the juice.

Time to Lose Your Bottle

It's not only food that gets cooked these days, but also the fruit and vegetable juices you see in shops. Remember, when we cook our food to death, that's exactly what has happened – the life has been blasted out. The same applies to our drinks. **All bottled, canned and carton juices and smoothies are cooked!** Even the '100 per cent', 'not from concentrate' ones are cooked. Cooked juices (or pasteurized, as they are more commonly referred to) are toxic (to greater and lesser degrees) to the body. It is extremely important you know this as I don't want you thinking you can simply replace my recommendations with some shop-bought varieties and have the same health success. Yes, you may still lose weight, but that is not my main goal here and it shouldn't be yours. The main goal is to *Juice Yourself Slim* in a *healthy* and *balanced* way.

Shop-bought juices still contain vitamins and minerals but to a *much* lesser degree than freshly extracted, raw and very much alive juices, and they are no longer properly balanced.

Freshly extracted juices are in a different league to shop-bought ones.

As you will be replacing some meals with juices and smoothies it is essential you don't simply have bottled or carton versions. The initial seven-day Launch Programme and the Juice Yourself Slim *for Life* programme have been carefully balanced nutritionally with natural, live, freshly extracted juices in mind. You can still have shop-bought juices from time to time, as some are very good, but freshly extracted juices are in a different league. In fact, if there were a 'juice league' in the same way as we have a football league, it would look something like this:

PREMIER DIVISION
Freshly extracted juice and fresh smoothies made with **organic** ingredients. Made either at home or at a very good organic juice bar (they are rare).

CHAMPIONSHIP DIVISION
Freshly extracted juice and fresh smoothies made with any ripe fresh ingredients, but washed thoroughly, made either at home or in juice bars. (Please see notes on 'juice bars' on page 162 as not all are as healthy and as 'ethical' as they appear.)

DIVISION 2
One hundred per cent organic, not from concentrate juices and smoothies in shop fridge section with short sell-by date made with **100 per cent pure fruit and/or veg**. Not from concentrate.

DIVISION 3

Non organic — one hundred per cent fresh fruit or veg juices and smoothies, *not from concentrate*.

DIVISION 4

One hundred per cent juices and smoothies made from concentrate.

NON-LEAGUE DIVISION

Any juice containing added sugars, artificial sweeteners, flavourings, preservatives or other additives. These are extremely harmful to the natural balance of the body. These juices are *very* common so you need to look at the label in detail. There are many 'juice cons' out there and I will cover them later.

in a Juicy League of Their Own

You will notice that even 100 per cent, non organic not from concentrate fruit and vegetable juices and smoothies are in Division 3! You will also notice that there isn't a Division 1. The reason for this is simple: freshly extracted juice is in a completely different league to any other juice or smoothie, not only in taste and aesthetics but, more importantly, in pure 'live' nutrition too. In reality we have no idea just how far apart they are.

When you change the molecular structure of nature's foods to the extent of pasteurization you destroy a great deal more than a few vitamins and minerals. Estimates suggest that up to 30 per cent of many natural plant foods defies scientific analysis. Personally, I think it's far and above that percentage. This means that even scientists agree they do not fully know what is in an apple! An apple a day may keep the doctor away, but science can't tell you why. This is because no matter how arrogant we are as humans, sometimes things are way bigger than us and we have to accept nature has provided the perfect fuel for us, fuel we cannot improve upon. When you interfere with the natural nutritional balance of nature's finest liquid fuel – a balance designed to feed, heal and protect – it relegates a liquid with premiership capabilities to a much lower division.

We will never improve on nature, and nothing is more naturally effective for the treatment and prevention of disease than freshly extracted ORGANiC juices and smoothies.

This is why you can't take one element of, say, an apple, carrot or orange, add some synthetic chemicals and expect it to have the same effect as the combination nature designed for us. All the chemical elements in the 'live' liquid fuel encased within the fibres of fruits and vegetables work synergistically – together – as one. We will never improve on nature, and nothing is more naturally effective against the treatment and prevention of disease – and, of course, 'global wobbling' – than freshly extracted *organic* juices and smoothies.

Too Much Knowledge …

We regard our species as the most intelligent on earth, yet it is the only species that suffers from this disease known as 'obesity'. We know more about nutrition, have more studies, more books and more pills, yet we are still killing ourselves with our forks. You may well find a few isolated exceptions in the wild with regard to disease, but while some of you are arguing the toss, your inner sanctum is looking more like Baghdad than Mauritius. I know many people with degrees – even in the area of nutrition – who dismiss the 'wild animal' and 'raw' argument, but whichever way you cut it, you won't ever see a gorilla tossing anything on a barbecue! And while the issue is being debated, we are getting sicker and fatter than ever.

I'm not against cooked food. **i LOVE** a cooked meal and I love dinner parties. I am simply illustrating the importance of the raw factor, or X factor if you will. Unlike many who advocate the power of 'raw', I am far from evangelical about it. I don't want people to adopt a raw-only diet or become a 'juicearian' (if there is such a thing). I simply want people to look at both the scientific and what is deemed 'anecdotal' evidence and do what they instinctively know is best for them.

The Everlasting Light Bulb

I remember back in the 1980s seeing a market stall selling 'everlasting light bulbs' for £5 each. At the time, when your average light bulb was about 30p, £5 was a hell of a lot. However, these were everlasting and, as such, a bargain at the price. They sold, as you can imagine, like hot cakes. Now, your average light bulb lasts for about eight months. Guess how long they were there selling their wares? Three months. They weren't just selling them at East Street Market in southeast London, but simultaneously at many markets across the UK. People saw them week after week and assumed they were genuine, but after eight months the bulbs had gone, as had the sellers.

Equally, it takes many, many years for disease to manifest itself as something we can recognize and name. This means 'experts' can say almost what they like. By the time anything does happen, opinions will have changed. Those government 'experts' who stated nutritional, disease or drug facts which are later proved wrong will, like the everlasting light bulb sellers, be long gone.

This doesn't matter so much with the light bulb as you have lost £5 and some pride for falling for such a trick, but when it comes to your health and one and only life, listening to the wrong people can be very costly indeed. Science and the medical profession have been wrong before, as have many in the 'alternative' field. This is why I urge people not to simply listen or buy into what I or anyone is saying, but to ask 'does it make sense to *me?*' If it makes sense – *intuitive common sense* – then roll with it. If it doesn't – don't. Let's not forget that many in the medical profession once said baby formula was much better than breast milk and that cigarettes were great for many things, including relaxation. No, I'm not kidding, relaxation – nicotine is a bloody stimulant!

If an 'expert' says powdered milk is better than breast milk and that sticking an object containing 4,000 different chemicals into a hole in your head and setting fire to it is in any way good, don't listen. You may think you would never believe such things whoever was suggesting them. But years ago people did believe things simply because a doctor and science had said it was the truth. Believe it or not, homosexuality was once classified as a disease too!

When do you think the following statement was written?

'Even though just ten years ago we thought we knew the proper treatments of illness, we now know just how little we knew back then ... with these revolutionary breakthroughs in technology, virtually all illness and disease should be wiped out in America within the next ten years. We are on the verge of entering a phase where a person will never be sick. And if you do get sick, your doctor will be able to cure you of your illness in a matter of days. We have virtually reached the pinnacle of medical knowledge.'

Last week? Last year? Nope – try 1902. Yes, in 1902 the words above were written to hail the end of all disease and to laugh at how little was known a decade before. The people who wrote such nonsense are, like the everlasting light bulb folk, long gone. Disease is virtually unknown in the wild, a place free of medical science which relies solely on nature's food to heal, protect and nurture. Clearly we are not in the wild and *at times* medical intervention is *extremely* important. However, I am simply illustrating that the fluid contained within nature's plants designed for human fuel is far more effective at the prevention of disease than any patented drug can possibly be. I also believe nature's fuel should play a major role in the healing of disease, *especially* after medical treatments or alongside them.

The fluid contained within nature's plants designed for human fuel is far more effective at the prevention of disease than any patented drug can possibly be.

Caring for Your Inner Environment

According to the American Cancer Society, it can take 20 years to build some types of cancer. *Prevention* is of paramount importance and yet we only appear to get help and advice *after* we already have obvious signs of the disease.

All diseases are caused by chemicals. All diseases can be cured by chemicals. All chemicals used by the body except for the oxygen we breathe, and the water which we drink, are taken through food. if we only knew enough, all diseases could be prevented and could be cured through proper nutrition. As tissues become damaged, they lack the chemicals for good nutrition. They tend to become old. They lack what i call 'tissue integrity'. There are people of forty whose brains and arteries are senile. if we could help the tissues repair themselves by correcting nutritional deficiencies, we can make age wait.

— Tom Spies MD who was honoured by the American Medical Association for his contribution to the healing art through his work with foods

This is why the second you stop ingesting chemical poisons and start to furnish the body with the vital nutritional chemicals required for optimum health, the many symptoms of disease improve or dissolve altogether. In other words, the very second you start to take care of your inner environment, your external environment – skin, hair, nails, body shape and so on – begins to improve. This couldn't be better illustrated than in all the testimonials you have read in this book and the tens of thousands we have received over the years. Furnish the body with nature's finest organic green super fuel and magic occurs, especially when it comes to removing **EXCESS FAT**.

The very second you start to take care of your inner environment, your external environment — skin, hair, nails, body shape and so on — begins to improve.

‘Hi there :o)

Well, here i am on Day 8 of your juice programme … and what a fantastic week!

i just stepped on the scales and found i have lost an amazing 10lbs!!! JOY! i weighed in at 15st 2lbs last Saturday and a very sad 37-year-old man i was too … but to find that after just seven easy-juicy days i'm almost a stone lighter at 14st 4lbs. Amazed, overjoyed, thrilled — there aren't really any words, are there?

STOP! i've just reread what i've written … 14st 4lbs … weighed again to double-check … 12lbs not 10!!! i've had to come back to this email after realizing my calculations were wrong — i really have lost nearly a stone. 12lbs not 10?! Oh my God. it's a good job i'm sitting down :o) i'm telling everyone my good news and spreading the word — what a brilliant 'diet'.

Now i've calmed down i can inform you that right from Day 1 i have not felt hungry once … not once! My energy has gone up, i wake up feeling brilliant — no 'bed-head' syndrome, no tiredness — just refreshed and ready to get up and go. The detox headaches on Days 2 and 3 were pretty bad but i stuck in there. Saying that, it's been brilliant and here's to the next phase.

i suffer with iBS, and prior to going on the 'diet' i was having stomach cramps and bloating. These symptoms have not reared their ugly heads once this week. Another not too nice thing i noticed was that since reaching the 15st mark i'd been so sweaty! Yuk! i work in an office and wear a shirt and tie and i was forever checking under my arms for those nasty damp patches — so embarrassing in meetings. Later in the week — completely dry! i think it was due to me being so overweight and as i just got more uptight about it, it obviously made things worse. This week, though, i've been so relaxed, in such a great frame of mind — really calm and happy/contented with myself. Now i'm just so fired up to carry on with the next phase and discover what my next weigh-in will bring. it's such a massive boost to my confidence.

Anyway, there you have it — a little bit warts-and-all but i think honesty is best. Hope i haven't rambled on!

Many, many thanks to the Juice Master for inspiring me!
Mr C Brown 〕

Twelve pounds in eight days, no symptoms of IBS, no stomach cramps, no bloating, and he hasn't felt hungry once – not once! Why? Because if you are 'chemically short' your body will inevitably call for the chemicals it requires to feed itself, maintain health and prevent disease. We will know this as a feeling and thought of 'I'm hungry'. This is why before I started to flood my system with liquid fuel I was eating like a horse! No wonder I was fat. The more crap I ate, and the more chemically *short* I became, the hungrier I got. The hungrier I got the more I ate and the fatter I got. The fatter I got the more of me there was and the more fuel I needed just to maintain my bigger frame and fill my bigger stomach.

The majority of overweight people aren't 'pigs'; they are simply coming up chemically and nutritionally short. Once this man started to give his body the nutrition it had been crying out for, the less hunger he felt. This meant he didn't have a 'diet mentality', which occurs when you are fighting against trying to satisfy a hunger, but rather one of 'food freedom'. This is why it's possible to lose weight without dieting. Dieting is not about the food but the frame of mind. If you are constantly hungry and feel deprived all the time, you are 'on a diet'; if you don't and are excited about what you are doing, you're not. It's that simple. What's also interesting is the fact he used to perspire to the point of embarrassment, and after just a few days of pure juice and smoothies – dry as a bone.

Although you may well have picked up this book simply to *Juice Yourself Slim*, many aspects of your physical and mental wellbeing will improve way beyond just getting into your jeans or little black dress. My aim is not simply to help people slim, but to show exactly why juicing and keeping the inner environment as pollution-free as possible is of paramount importance to your mental and physical wellbeing, both now and in the future. To give you an even better idea of the level of importance I'm talking about, it's worth knowing that in the right environmental conditions, **cells can live forever in a laboratory**. If you take a cell and place it in fluid, the cell will create waster matter and toxins. However, studies have shown that as long as you clean that environment and continually get rid of the waste matter and toxins, the cells never age! **THAT'S HOW IMPORTANT YOUR ENVIRONMENT IS TO YOUR HEALTH AND LOOKS!**

> **There are twenty active vitamins needed by your body and seventeen minerals and trace elements. You can get them all in juices.**
>
> — Dr Bernard Jensen

What's even more wonderful is that there is a way to help both the inner *and* external environments at the same time. I mentioned at the start of this chapter that we know global warming is happening, but it is far from clear what causes it. The jury is still very much out (at the time of writing) as to whether the problem is caused by us or would simply be happening anyway. I also mentioned that because we don't know, and given that the health of the planet could be at stake, it's nice to know that by following the *Juice Yourself Slim* way of life, you will inadvertently be doing more to save the external environment than if you walked everywhere and skipped all flights. Don't believe me? Read on.

One Big Meaty Global Problem

By simply cutting down the amount of meat and dairy in your diet – or cutting them out completely – you will be doing more to save the planet than you might think. But you won't hear that from the Al Gore camp, and it appears the UK government isn't exactly shouting about this easy solution. In a 408-page report entitled 'Livestock's Long Shadow', United Nations scientists declared that: 'Meat and dairy animals are the second biggest cause of greenhouse gases at 18% (at time of writing) compared to 13.5% from all of the world's different modes of transport combined.' Let me emphasize this piece of stark reality:

Meat and dairy cause more greenhouse gases than all the world's modes of transport combined.

The science in this case really couldn't be clearer. I don't wish to labour the point, but it's worth hammering home – **COMBINED!** That's **ALL** the vehicles in the world. Think about that for a second. Scientists at the University of Chicago showed that a typical American meat-eater is responsible for nearly 1.5 tons more carbon dioxide a year than a vegan, and the figure is no doubt similar here in the UK. On top of this, according to a UN report, raising animals for food is '**one of the top two or three most significant contributors to the most serious environmental problems, at every scale from local to global**'. Almost half of the water and 80 per cent of the agricultural land in the US are used to raise animals for food. **You need 10 times the land to feed a meat-eater than you do a vegetarian, and even less for a vegan**.

On top of this massive pollution to our environment caused by meat and dairy, these foods don't exactly do much for a clean, healthy, vibrant and slim body either. Yes, Mr Atkins may well have got millions consuming an enormous amount of meat and dairy in the name of 'slim', but along with a slim body came breath straight from Satan's bottom, lethargy and an extremely acidic system, which caused plenty of problems for many of Atkins' followers. Eating *nothing* but meat may well make you thin, but will do jack to make you truly healthy. Drinking coffee and taking heroin will also make you thin!

Excess meat and dairy intake not only contributes to environmental sickness (if man is indeed the cause), but also our own. There have been many studies linking excess animal protein consumption to human sickness. Plus of course it is the cause of its very own disease – Mad Cow. Our systems require high water content, chemically rich, nutrient-packed foods – meat doesn't exactly fit this bill. As for dairy, drinking the 'food' of another animal designed to transform a 200lb calf at birth to one of over 2,000lbs in just two years is bound to bring its own challenges. It is now reported that up to 70 per cent of us are becoming 'dairy intolerant'. I doubt if we will ever reach a stage where most of society is 'broccoli intolerant' or 'avocado intolerant', do you? Many are dairy intolerant simply because it's not blooming normal to consume the milk of another creature, *especially* after weaning age. We are, after all, the only mammals who continue drinking milk after we have been weaned, but we drink the milk of a completely different species, one with four stomachs! Why do you think dairy ever became one of the major food groups? Anything to do with a vested interest between the dairy industry and the government? Again, just a thought, but do you remember the subsidized butter mountains?

Choosing a Greener Diet

I realize this all sounds a tad evangelical and I would forgive you for thinking I am part of some 'animal rights' movement, and that I'm here not to juice you slim but to try to put you on some kind of guilt trip to save animals or the earth. The reality is that, despite being a 'vegan' for a couple of years, I now like a bit of cheese as much as the next person and recently I've even indulged in some organic chicken. I am also extremely sceptical about the whole external environment argument: when I say 'sceptical', I mean I don't believe it at all. That doesn't mean I don't take this subject seriously. I believe recycling is extremely important, not because of this apparent man-made global warming, but simply because we'll have nothing left to sustain us if we use everything up unnecessarily. I also know that our bodies are amazing and can deal with small amounts of anything without any long-term damage, so feel free to have your cheese and meat from time to time, if that's what floats your boat.

All I am saying is that as excess animal protein has been well-documented as causing problems to our internal environment – as well as now being recognized as a *major* contributing factor to external environment pollution – doesn't the easiest solution seem to be to cut down on your intake or cut it out altogether? For most readers, meat and dairy will be a taste and lifestyle choice, not a matter of life or death. For some people in the world it is, but here in our world, it just isn't. We are being asked to make many sacrifices in the name of the 'environment', yet unlike not using our cars or going on planes, we can all do this without any real disruption to our lives. The side-effect is simply a healthy and slimmer body and a cleaner environment. It's a no-brainer really. On top of this, if we did apply this simple solution we would also help save billions of animals from being killed each year in the name of 'nugget', 'dog' and 'burger'. So a good thing all round methinks.

There is no doubt – and I would lay money on it – that when 15,000 people flew to the United Nations Conference on Climate Change in Bali in 2007(yes **FLEW,** many on private jets), meat was very much on the menu. I fear the irony of pushing out the annual CO2 of an African country to the tune of 100,000 tons of carbon dioxide with air travel while munching on a T-bone passed them by!

However, this book is not about 'saving the planet' but rather saving yourself. Saving yourself from the mental and physical discomfort of being overweight or obese. Saving yourself from the embarrassment of not being able to get into a swimming costume in public, or wearing the clothes you want on a regular basis. It's about saving yourself from the frustration of not being as active as you would like to be and and, of course, it's about saving yourself from the sheer nightmare of serious disease, now and in the future. With two out of three of us *guaranteed* to end up with either heart disease or cancer, we aren't as invincible as we like to believe. Which is why, above all, it is essential that sooner rather than later you start investing in ...

5

The Finest Health Insurance in the World

If you have seen Michael Moore's documentary *SiCKO*, you will know that health care in the US is somewhat different to that in the UK. You would also think after watching it that here in the UK everything is perfect, that we don't possess waiting lists and that people are seen within 20 minutes when in A & E – which is somewhat far from the truth.

The documentary drew attention to the sad state of affairs in the US when it comes to health care and, more importantly, health insurance. In the US (at the time of writing), unless you have health insurance you're screwed. There are many cases where you will be turned away without treatment unless you can show proof of your health insurance, no matter how sick you are.

Not everyone qualifies for health insurance either. If there is the slightest possibility you may get sick at any point soon, expect to see the word **DENiED** plastered all over your application. Knowing you don't have health cover brings its own stress, and stress is one of the largest contributors to ill health there is.

The situation on the health care front in the US isn't good, but then – despite how it may look in *SiCKO* – it isn't that great here either. I also love this illusion that we have 'free' health care in the UK. Unless I am mistaken, don't we all pay National Insurance? Isn't it our money? I agree ours is a much, much better system than in the US, but let's not be deluded into thinking it's all hunky-dory. My mum went in to have a cyst the size of an orange removed from one of her ovaries when I was just 15. They removed the *wrong* flipping ovary and she has suffered ever since!

When I went into hospital covered in psoriasis and looking for a diagnosis I had dozens of student doctors all proding my semi-naked sore-covered body, guessing at what I had (yeah, nice!). One of the students said to the main physician, 'I think it's psoriasis,' to which he replied, 'NO.' This answer surprised me as I thought that's what it was. I was informed I actually had scabies and was told to cover myself in this nasty-smelling cream and leave it on for 48 hours. Forty-eight hours later I still had what was, in reality, psoriasis. No doubt you will know many horror stories yourself of people not exactly getting the level of treatment you would expect from a 21st-century health care system, one which we expect the world to follow.

Very Personal Health Care

I can understand Michael Moore's frustration with his health care system, and I can also understand the anger often generated by some of the health care in the UK, but a touch of personal responsibility wouldn't go amiss either. We are all quick to blame the NHS, and bitch and moan about what 'they' should be doing for us. As far as we are concerned, we have paid in and they should fix us if/when something goes wrong. Look at Michael Moore. If you haven't seen him, he is hardly the picture of health and vibrancy – in fact, he is a heart attack waiting to happen. No wonder he is concerned about the health care system and wants a state-run alternative. After all, he is probably going to have to spend a great deal on health insurance (if anyone will give it to him) and treatment any time soon. The point I am making is that while it's good to challenge the system and not simply put up with an unjust or failing health service, don't we all have a degree of personal responsibility?

National Breakdown Cover

We have an 'emergency breakdown' mentality when it comes to our health. I think this stems from other areas of our lives where this makes sense, such as with our cars. As long as we are a member of the AA or RAC, we don't need to drive with fear. If something does go wrong, we are usually just an hour away from assistance. The car is either fixed there and then, or towed to a garage for repairs. The worst possible scenario is a little inconvenience and perhaps a car pronounced 'dead on arrival' at the garage. Ths isn't a nice situation, but it's not life-threatening either. In no time at all we pick up another car and the whole thing is forgotten.

We simply cannot apply this same principle to our health. People think that if they have health insurance it's all okay. But in the same way that buying a great cook book doesn't make you Jamie Oliver, merely paying for private or national health care doesn't for one second make you healthy. Nor does it mean everything will be okay if something goes wrong due to the level of cover you have. If this vehicle gets pronounced 'dead on arrival', there's no nipping out to get another one with 'no down payment and 0 per cent interest' – the show's over!

I know some millionaires who would gladly swap every penny they have to turn the clock back and look after themselves differently. Money cannot buy you true health; you can only *do* health. Of course, not all disease is caused simply by someone not looking after themselves. We all know people who have eaten crap all their lives and done no exercise and lived a disease-free life. At the same time, we know many people who have eaten nothing but good foods, exercised daily and, yes, disease took hold and they died early. But once again this is very, *very* much the exception. Common sense tells us that if we regularly starve our cells of much needed nutrition and fail to help the body's natural cleaning system (the lymph system) to function properly, the huge chances are we will need some kind of health care.

This is why we can't simply get angry with the system *after* we get sick if we don't get the treatment we expect. Surely we have an obligation to help the system too? If hospitals were left for genuine cases of purely hereditary conditions and emergency accidents, we really would have the finest health care system in the world, and we would always be able to find a bed when one was needed. We are constantly asking, quite rightly, 'what are they doing'? But equally, ask yourself 'what the hell are you doing?'

Uncle Fred Syndrome

We all like to think that 'Uncle Fred' smoked, drank and ate crap yet lived till he was 150, but Uncle Freds are few and far between, and usually made up in order to justify overeating, smoking or drinking. When I smoked God-knows-how-many cigarettes daily, I concentrated on the news that a French woman had lived to the incredibly ripe old age of 119 yet had only stopped smoking when she was 115! This woman made front page news, yet the millions of smokers whose lungs collapse, whose legs have been removed and who have lung cancer seemingly weren't newsworthy. I conveniently chose to ignore them too. While it's true that not all smokers get lung cancer, over 90 per cent of people who do get lung cancer *are* smokers.

Exactly the same thing happens with food and fat. We constantly – whether consciously or subconsciously – look for people who eat and drink crap yet appear and are 'healthy'. Advertisers do it all the time. Get David Beckham, rather than Robbie Coltrane, to drink the heavily sugared and synthetic chemical-loaded Pepsi and you can easily send a clear message that this stuff is fine and dandy. Get the extremely beautiful Jennifer Aniston (okay, so I like her ... *a lot!*) rather than Rosanne Barr to eat some Ben and Jerry's on screen and it's easy to be deluded into thinking this stuff will keep you as slim as a rake.

We are constantly doing our own market research, on the lookout for people who can enable us to justify the mass pollution of our inner worlds. We are looking for people like Buster – the oldest working man in the UK at the time of writing – who drinks alcohol and eats mainly rubbish. Why do you think Buster is newsworthy? Because he is rare – bloody rare! We ignore the hundreds of millions of people who are dropping like flies from heart disease, stroke, cancer, diabetes, arthritis, and so the list goes on and on. Why? Why do we ignore this overwhelming evidence? Because many are 'addicted' and, as I have mentioned, we feel invincible. We have the 'it will never happen to us' mentality. But there is no question that if you play the junk, fat and no exercise Russian Roulette, it *will* most likely happen to you. The bottom line is you are *not* invincible.

People who cite the likes of 'Uncle Fred' also say, 'They got away with it' and 'It never caught up with them' and 'They had a disease-free life.' But take just smoking as an example. If someone manages to survive till they are 100 while smoking, it doesn't mean they got away with 'it' at all. They were still smokers, and every single day they suffered the slavery of that addiction. Every day they *had* to smoke. Every time they finished a meal at a restaurant they *had* to go outside and face Hurricane Gilbert. Every day they had to put up with the smell on their breath, their hair, their clothes. Each and every day they had to continue doing something they would rather be free of in an ideal world. Every day they were being controlled and dictated to. Every night they went to bed praying they would just wake up one day and not want a cigarette.

I know this because I used to smoke two to three packets of cigarettes a day, every day, for God knows how many years. I didn't stop smoking because I thought I'd get cancer – I reasoned that I could get run over by a bus the next week. I stopped smoking because it controlled me. I stopped smoking because my life was dictated to by these addictive little tubes of poison. I was always going to have a cigarette and do something, or I was going to do something and then have a cigarette. I was lucky in the end. I did get away with it – I managed to stop *and* I didn't get lung cancer. Those who smoke till the day they die, regardless of what age that is, did *not* get away with it, even if they didn't get cancer. 'IT' is not the disease that may or may not happen. '**iT**' is the daily problems being a smoker creates – that in itself is a disease. A long-drawn-out and often painful disease which may lead to one of the BIG diseases in the end.

Equally, if someone is overweight and addicted to junk*ie* and chemically loaded foods all their lives but somehow manages to live till they are 100, they also didn't get away with 'it'. Being overweight and having certain foods control you is the same as being a smoker in that it brings its own *daily* challenges. I didn't slim down just because I thought I might get heart disease or cancer one day. Once again, my mindset of 'life's too short' often prevents me from thinking such things. No, I slimmed down simply because I hated how being fat was affecting my *daily* existance. I hated my body, my energy levels, the fact I was a guy and had flipping breasts! I hated the way I looked in clothes and not in clothes. I also hated being a slave to chemically addictive 'food'. I hated stuffing myself and feeling like shit afterwards. I hated the fact that I was being controlled by artificial chemicals on a daily basis.

If someone does survive a fat life for 100 years, they didn't get away with it! 'IT' is the daily mental and physical nightmare of being overweight, of being fat and lethargic and hating the way you look and feel. It's the nightmare of not having that energetic mental and physical spark that makes you want to suck the juice out of each and every short day we have on this planet. It's the frustration of wanting to burst out of bed all guns blazing, but not being able to do so.

So, yes, some people do survive for years despite being overweight or smoking, but they are *rare* and they don't truly live to their capacity. They also spend a large part of their lives hating their situation. If you are reading this book you are clearly 'alive', but the mere fact you are reading a book of this nature (unless you are doing so for research) means you are clearly not 'getting away with it' either. You are upset when you eat crap and upset if you feel you can't – it's a seeming no-win situation.

Even if you don't suffer the daily mental and physical struggle of being overweight and lethargic, taking action *now* in order to avoid the horrific nightmare of living through a degenerative disease is still extremely wise. Yes, it is true you may not get heart disease or cancer or God knows what else, but there is a two out of three chance you will. It's funny how people do the lottery with odds of fourteen million to one, and think it will happen to them, and yet a two in three chance like this and they somehow believe it won't be them. Those kinds of odds suck, especially when we are talking about your one and only life. So why risk it for the sake of a couple of fresh green juices a day?

Put it in the Bank – NOW!

By having a couple of nutritionally rich juices a day we are getting perhaps the finest form of genuine nutrition available to us in our polluted, over-farmed and conglomerate food world.

By juicing yourself slim, or more specifically juicing yourself to health, you will be supplying your one and only health bank account with a daily dose of much needed credit. None of us are perfect on the food and drink front (yes, even me!) but by having a couple of nutritionally rich, chemically balanced, pure, organic (where possible) juices a day we are at least getting perhaps the finest form of genuine nutrition available to us in our polluted, over-farmed and conglomerate food world. In fact, it's worth knowing that in the 21st century

You will NOT get the same level of nutrition by eating fruit and veg as you will when you juice them.

And that even includes organic fruit and veg!

To top up your nutritional bank account and keep it fully in the black, freshly extracted juices are far more essential than people think. At this stage you may find that hard to believe, and if you are in the medical or dietetic world you may well find it impossible to believe. However, there are two fundamental reasons why I believe this is so:

- Most of us have an extremely battered and not fully efficient digestive system, making it almost impossible for us to gain maximum nutrition from solid food.
- Most fruit and veg in the 21st century is coming up nutritionally short.

The idea behind juicing is to furnish our systems with the 'live' chemicals required for optimum health without burdening our digestive system. After years of eating the wrong foods, our digestive system is already tired and often clogged and sluggish. This makes it virtually impossible to get the full nutritional value from a piece of fruit or a vegetable simply by eating it. The body is, essentially, just one big juice extractor. When we eat an apple, all the body tries to do is extract the juice from the fibre. All of the vitamins, minerals, enzymes and co-factors are contained within the juice – not the fibre. **Fibre does not and cannot feed the body.** If your internal 'juice extractor' isn't working well, it won't extract the maximum amount of juice. By eating fruit or veg you are simply *hoping* you will get the levels of nutrition required to give you excellent health as opposed to *knowing for certain* that you will if you drink the freshly extracted juice.

You are not what you eat. You are what you managed to absorb.

However, even if you have the best digestive system on earth and your internal juicer is okay, you still can't get the level of nutrition your body needs by simply eating the food. This is because our food is not what it once was. These days it is dramatically depleted of essential vitamins and minerals, so we need to consume much more to reach our true chemical nutritional needs. This isn't always possible due the body's natural digestive restrictions. For example, the body wasn't designed to eat three apples at exactly the same time (we couldn't fit them in our mouth for one!). However, it takes at *least* three of today's often 'polluted' non-organic apples to reach the same level of nutrition as one grown in dense mineral-rich soil with little chemical fertilizers, pesticides and fungicides back in the 1950s. So although you may not be able to eat three apples at once, you can extract the juice from the apples and easily drink them. This is why 'live' liquid is such an efficient and delicious way to guarantee a solid health care system.

Organic Health Care Versus 'Normal' Health Care

A study published in the *Journal of Agriculture and Food Industry* in 2003 showed that organically grown berries contained 58 per cent more polyphenols than those grown conventionally. As far back as 1993, a study showed that over a two-year period organic foods contained up to four times as many trace minerals, 13 times more selenium and 20 times more calcium and magnesium than commerically produced foods. And that's what we know about. Who knows how much of the X factor was lost?

However, even though organic produce has many times the nutritional value of non-organic produce – and even though it is free of chemical fertilizers that are incredibly toxic to our systems – you still can't get your full quota by eating food alone. Due to over-farming, our soil is depleted of essential minerals. This means it is virtually impossible to meet your body's true health insurance needs by eating the produce alone, even when it is organic.

To put your mind at rest, all of this doesn't mean we're screwed if don't juice organic, or that eating fruit will give us nothing. There is clearly *plenty* of nutrition even in non-organic fruits and vegetables, and more in organic. You would also still get a degree of much needed nutrition by eating them and not juicing. I am simply explaining why juicing is more important today than it has ever been in order to get the **FULL** nutritional value and **FULL** health care protection.

What is clear is that people don't eat enough fruit and vegetables of any kind. So although people often ask, 'Why don't we just eat it?' I can only say, 'I don't know why, but we don't!' And that's the truth. It is estimated that the average person in the UK eats around 5 per cent 'live raw' food a week – the rest is processed in some way. That's **5 PER CENT!**

If you don't believe me, next time you are in a supermarket just look at people's trollies. If you see even one with as much as 30 per cent 'live' foods you have seen the exception. And let's not forget that much of the 'live' food you see in the trolly will soon be sitting on 'death row', waiting to be cooked.

i LOVE, LOVE, LOVE juicing. You can drink even 10 fruits and vegetables at once in their raw form and get the maximum amount of nutritional investment from each one.

So any amount of juicing, even if the fruit and veg are covered in chemical fertilizers, will be a dose of much needed investment for your health. I would never get the level of nutrition I receive now unless I juiced, whether organic or 'normal'. As good as something like raw broccoli is for you, I would never get excited at the thought of eating a load of it. However, I get the water-rich, nutrient-packed goodness of raw broccoli simply by juicing it with some apples, maybe a bit of pineapple, a tad of ginger and a small amount of lemon to give it some zing!

Personally, I hate raw vegetables, always have done. I like a salad now and again, but even that took some gettting used to. This is why **i LOVE, LOVE, LOVE** juicing. You can drink even 10 fruits and vegetables at once in their raw form and get the maximum amount of nutritional investment from each one without having to eat them raw. Juicing has only just come into the 21st century, and given the state of our food and the need to access as much nutrition as possible from fresh produce, the timing couldn't have been better.

When it comes to health insurance, nutrition plays a major role. However, it's not everything. In order to give yourself the best possible chance of avoiding the major players in the disease world – and to make certain you *do* get away with 'IT' – it's time to start …

6

Exercising Your God-given Right to Better Health Insurance

Love it or hate it, your body was designed to move. Not shuffle along, I mean **MOVE!** I believe this aspect is even more important than raw nutrition when it comes to health care investment. I once read this in a weight-loss book: '… doing exercise is like driving your car simply in order to put petrol in …'. This implied that the *only* benefit of exercising was to burn fuel. The author's point was why bother exercising just to make yourself require more fuel? Why not simply put in less fuel according to your needs and skip exercise altogether? Sounds like common sense but wrong on many levels. I believe he even cited an example of 'snails not rushing around yet not being overweight' in his book too, suggesting that you don't need to exercise to lose weight. I fear the fact that snails are moving about with their entire house on their back was missed by the author.

The car analogy is flawed in several respects, none more so than our bodies were designed to move for reasons other than simply to burn fuel. When we move our body aerobically (with air) we effectively power up our natural cleaning system – the lymph system. You have around four times more lymph fluid in your body than you do blood. However, whereas your blood has a perfectly good pump – your heart – your lymph fluid relies on breathing. It is true that without exercise your lymph system still functions, but to a lesser degree. Our cells are constantly regenerating – billions of cells have just died in your body right this second. The good news is that billions of cells have also rejuvenated themselves. Where do all the dead cells end up? In the lymph system. This makes us feel tired and sluggish, and is one of the reasons we often feel a great deal more tired after we have been sitting down for a long time than if we have just been for a walk. When you walk, run, swim and so on, you are firing up your lymph 'pump' and helping your body to eliminate toxins. Once the toxins are released you feel lighter, mentally sharper, more awake and usually – and somewhat ironically – *less* hungry.

There have been many times when, at the end of a day, I have felt extremely hungry and tired. I have the 'gym or food?' debate in my head, and many times the gym wins. When it does I **ALWAYS** feel more awake and less hungry than when I went in. Why? Because I sweated out a load of toxins which were causing lethergy, tiredness and hunger. Tiredness and hunger are often very similar feelings and it can often be hard to distinguish what the body actually wants. Often the body is simply craving a good blast of oxygen and some water. About an hour after the gym I am *nicely* hungry, my metabolism is still going strong and I always enjoy my food. I never have the feeling of 'I wish I hadn't done that' afterwards, regardless of what I have just eaten.

The other difference is that when you drive your car, the car doesn't get an endorphin rush! Doing a form of daily exercise not only helps to clean the lymph system, making us feel light, it also releases happy brain chemicals called endorphins. These make us feel good, and when we feel good we are much less inclined to succumb to emotional eating. Driving your car doesn't improve its body shape and inner and outer strength either. Exercise tones you up, both internally and externally. It's essential for the prevention of osteoporosis; it helps to strengthen the heart muscle, increases oxygen to the cells, stimulates the metabolism and reduces stress. A slim and toned body also feels bloody good, and a car – unless your name is Herbie – doesn't have feelings either!

When you walk, run or swim, you are helping your body to eliminate toxins. Once the toxins are released you feel lighter, mentally sharper, more awake and usually LESS hungry.

Movement = Life

There is no question that exercise is absolutely necessary on both a mental and physical level in order to reach the land of the slim, fit and healthy. There is also no question that a daily dose of exercise will do just as much as, if not more than, the right fuel in terms of investment into your personal health insurance. It is also the number-one key ingredient to bringing life into your life. When you move you feel alive. After all, if you are not moving whatsoever, that is called **DEATH!** The more you move, the more alive you feel.

However, like anything, you can get too much of a good thing. Too much exercise can cause excess free radical damage and, depending on what type of exercise you do, can cause injuries. Free radicals are quashed by antioxidants, and you will be pleased to know that the *Juice Yourself Slim* lifestyle is loaded with antioxidants. This means that if you do become a gym bunny and work out like a mad person, at least you are safe in the knowledge that nature's 'police force' will be on hand to take care of any free radical riots taking place. When I hit the gym I often make myself a nice juice, pour it into a flask and drink it in the sauna afterwards. Any free radicals which may have built up are soon neutralized. At this stage you may think that exercising too much won't be an issue for you, but once those endorphins are released on a daily basis, it can be addictive!

Try Rebounding

There are many ways in which you can move your body to help your lymph system, create an endorphin high and rev up your metabolism. However, I don't feel the need to patronize you by giving you a list. You would have to have been stuck on the planet Zog not to know at least a dozen ways in which you can exercise your body on a daily basis. I do love it when an expert suggests, 'Take the stairs and not the lift' or 'Doing the housework burns X amount of calories'. Come on, be honest. When you hear this isn't there a part of you which thinks, 'Oh bog off!' (or words to that effect)? So I won't make any stupidly obvious suggestions. Instead I would just like to share with you one of the easiest ways to work out several times a day for short bursts at a time. This form of exercise is growing in popularity almost daily. You don't need to be a member of a gym, and unless you live in an upstairs flat (and don't get on with your downstairs neighbours) or in a little cottage with a very low ceiling, it can be done almost anywhere. It is rebounding (or jumping on a mini-trampoline) and according to NASA no less, it is **'the most efficient and effective exercise yet devised by man'.**

It has also been reported that, '… it is the only form of exercise that actually affects, in a positive way, every cell in the body simultaneously …' I feel this may be a little far-fetched as there must be at least one other type of exercise that also does this. However, rebounding and swimming are the only two exercises that work *every single muscle* in the body, without jarring the joints. Many people on my retreats are surprised at how much their *upper* body aches after their first time on one of these amazing pieces of equipment. It's particularly good for what's known as 'bingo wings'!

I have been using a mini-trampoline for 10 years. It's the one piece of exercise equipment that doesn't end up being used as a clothes hanger! The main reason for that is because it's fun – a fairly unique concept when it comes to exercise. Janey Lee Grace, author of the quite excellent *Imperfectly Natural Woman*, says: 'You simply cannot bounce on a mini-trampoline and not smile'. It's also a form of exercise you can do inside or out, at home or at work, in a garden, park or even on the beach, and it's easy to do for a short amount of time several times a day. You can also do it in a group high in the mountains of southern Turkey, watching one of the most spectacular sunsets in the world whilst listening to uplifting music. This is something I have created at my retreats and it's my single favourite group exercise, especially in that setting. Granted, boucing in your home may not be quite the same, but with a blast of good music it's extremely uplifting. What's more, you can get a support bar with many good mini-trampolines, which means virtually anyone of any age can get the benefits of this often under-rated exercise. You can also put two mini-trampolines side by side and take it up a level!

In terms of your personal health insurance, *any* form of exercise is one of the best investments you can make, and is essential in the over-all 'slim and healthy for life' picture. People think of exercise as a means to an end instead of finding something that stimulates them, some-thing that becomes part of their daily life, something that really juices them into action. I used to hate exercise, but it is funny what happens after a short period of habit building. I even ran the New York Marathon in 2007, when only a few years ago I couldn't even run a bath, and the only marathon I was interested in was the one going down my throat! It was one of the most exhilarating times I have ever had on this planet. Crowds of people lining the streets of New York on a sunny November day, cheering, handing out bananas and water, and high-fiving you all the way. What a way to see a city. This is the kind of experience that regular physical movement can give you.

ANY form of exercise is one of the best investments you can make, and is essential in the overall 'slim and healthy for life' picture.

Remember, unlike a car, your body is running all the time and it was designed to move for many more reasons than simply to burn the fuel you put in. And unlike a car, you can't simply rely on some external breakdown service to pick up the pieces if anything goes wrong due to lack of exercise.

Movement is a Gift – Use It or Lose It

We take physical movement for granted, so much so that many people can't be bothered to move. Movement, however, is a true gift, and those who have lost this gift would give anything to get it back. If you can move, **MOVE!** The more you don't move the more you run the risk of losing the gift altogether. If, for example, I jump on a mini-trampoline every day, there won't ever be a day when I won't be able to do it unless I get injured in some way. My body is conditioned to expect me to do it and I will have no problem. Conversely, if you sit on a settee for years you will eventually seize up. Your muscles waste away, your bones become brittle and your cardio capacity reduces to meet its needs. You literally lose your ability and gift to move.

Exercise, or physical movement, is so, so, so much more than doing a bit to lose some weight. It is the very essence of feeling alive and protecting ourselves from the absolute nightmare of not being able to move in the future. When you start to *Juice Yourself Slim* and begin moving your body as part of that process, whatever you do – don't stop!

Health Care Gone Wild

In the wild, health care is simple. Animals eat the foods designed for their species by nature, and they move on a consistent basis – that's it! The natural chemicals within these 'live' foods help to nurture, heal and protect, and exercise helps to 'pump' out excess toxicity within the body. There's not a Bupa or Specsavers in the wild, and yet disease as we know it and poor eyesight or blindness isn't an issue. There's no 'waiting list' in the wild either, other than waiting to see if they can get hold of this amazing and nurturing 'live' food – a problem we are extremely fortunate not to have.

Every one of us has access to 'live' foods every day. We can easily furnish our accounts daily, top up our health insurance and reap the massive mental and physical rewards that come with it. Every one of us can invest in a 21st-century juicer or dust off the one hiding in the cupboard.

If you think you can't afford it – rubbish! People invest in alcohol (to the tune of £100,000 in the average drinker's life) and in cigarettes (the average one-pack-a-day smoker will spend over £65,000). They invest in things like Sky TV and meals out. So the chances are, if you are committed, you can easily get a juicer.

Every one of us (unless we have a severe disability) can also find the time and inclination to move on a regular basis. You don't need a gym membership or even a piece of exercise equipment if money really is an issue. A pair of trainers and a park or beach is all that's needed. If you have a beach nearby you don't even need the trainers.

The problem is we are good at talking about a healthy lifestyle but not so good at doing anything about it. We all want the rewards but don't want to do what it takes to get them. I know an amazing number of people who say they are concerned about things like E numbers and the amount of salt and sugar in everyday foods while smoking a fag, eating a doughnut and washing it down with a Coke.

We are now in a blame culture, so if we get sick or fat it's always someone else's fault. We blame it on things like 'our genes' (even if we have zero evidence to back that up), our hormones, having children to look after, not having the time due to work and home commitments, and even books. Yes, I know many, many people who blame their state of health and fatness on a book. I wish I was kidding, but I have had letters myself from people who said, 'I read your book, I lost weight but now I am fat again. Your programme doesn't work and the book was a waste of money.' It's amazing how some people will blame anything other than themselves.

'Diets' are usually the culprit: 'the diet failed' or 'the diet was rubbish'. It never seems to occur to us that perhaps, just perhaps, we might actually have something to do with it. People go on a diet because they are fat and indeed getting fatter by the week. They lose some weight on the diet, struggle and throw in the towel after a short while only to gain the weight and more back again. They then blame the diet for their additional pounds. What they fail to see is that they were gaining weight *before* the diet. They then come off it and pick up where they left off. Surprise, shock and horror! They gain weight again. But it's not the fact they went on a particular diet that caused the problem. It's the fact they went back to eating and drinking all the same crap in exactly the same way that caused the problem in the first place.

The harsh reality is that the only way to make a disease-free existance more likely – and not to end up on the 'surgeon's slab' – is to take your health insurance into your own hands. You cannot put it in the hands of an insurance company or even the state. All they can do is try to fix the mess *you* have, in all likelihood, created yourself. It's no good bitching about the system if you aren't willing to do your bit to help yourself.

Health Care DiY-style

From all the research I know about at the time of writing, it's clear that the *only* way to assure excellent health care cover is to take personal responsibility and do a touch of **DiY** – Drink It Yourself – while making sure you are moving your body. The main problem is most people tend to read a book like this, get a 'boost' and decide to take some responsibility, only to come crashing back down at some point in the future. My aim, above all else, is to stop this cycle for good and shift you from a short success mentality to one of lifelong success. It is simply the difference between ...

7

Changing Rooms versus Grand Designs

This chapter will make the difference between juicing yourself slim and healthy *for life* and juicing yourself slim *for a month* – so if you are tempted to skip it and just do the programme, don't! You have read this far, and if you are tempted to cut corners at this stage, it probably reflects a pattern. As I expressed at the start, laying the right mental foundations is the key to true slimming and health success. This chapter is one of the most important for tapping into a frame of mind that will make the whole process of getting slim and staying slim incredibly easy.

Laying the right mental foundations is the key to true slimming and health success.

Did you ever see the television programme *Changing Rooms*? The idea was simple. As the name suggests, two people living in two separate houses got the opportunity to help their neighbour transform a room in their home in just 48 hours with the help of design and build experts – usually with a budget of around £500. The programme ended with both neighbours being blindfolded before the all important 'revelation'. This was the moment when they saw what their neighbour – along with the experts and a truck-load of MDF – had done to their room.

As the blindfold came off, reactions ranged from delight to anger, usually with an expression of disbelief which silently read, 'What the f*** have you done to my house!' Even some of those who were happy with their new look found that their euphoria was short lived. The producers of *Changing Rooms Revisited* (when they went back six months later) probably wish they had thought a little more before deciding to go ahead with that follow-up programme as there were a few people who were very unhappy with the quality of the renovations that had been made.

Conversely, have you ever seen the television show *Grand Designs*? Here the programme follows a couple or individual throughout the entire journey of either building their own home or converting a unique building (like a water mill) into a spectacular living space. Unlike *Changing Rooms*, the journey is often long and usually involves extremely difficult obstacles. However, the end product is generally of amazing quality, a place of beauty and something to be truly proud of. They create a place where they *love* to live, where they *want* to live – a place which excites them, which won't fall apart after a couple of months.

Changing DIETS versus GRAND DESIGNS

Juice Yourself Slim, like *Grand Designs*, is all about creating something truly magnificent. Something that will last. Something to be proud of. It's about creating a light, energy-driven and totally juiced body and mind. A body that you are proud of. A body that makes you feel mentally alive and sexy! A body that enables you to truly live as opposed to simply survive. Once you tap into a Grand Design approach to your fitness and health, you feel excited from the start because you know you are about to create something of lasting magnitude.

However, there will be some who – despite everything they have read – will still do just the first seven days, get into their jeans or little black dress for the party and forget it. These people will soon gain weight again, and before they know where they are they will be looking for the next 'new' diet on the block. This is the 'Changing Diets' approach. 'Fat fluctuaters' go through this pattern all the time. They feel it's easier to cut corners in their bid to the slim life, only to find, like *Changing Rooms*, it all soon starts to fall apart.

There is a big difference between not wanting to be fat and wanting to be slim. They may sound the same but they are worlds apart.

A Changing Diet person tends to focus on what they don't want and has no real vision for what they do want. They are so busy trying to 'move away from' **FAT** as opposed to 'move towards' **SLIM,** that they continue in the same fat/slim … *ish*/fat spiral. There is a big difference between not wanting to be fat and wanting to be slim. They may sound the same but they are worlds apart.

The Fat Pressure Level

We all have what I call a 'fat' or 'health' pressure level. It's different for all of us but it's there. It's a level of fat or unhealthiness we aren't willing to go beyond. It's the desperation and deep remorse you experience when, once again, you have allowed yourself to get to this stage. It's the feeling that you would genuinely give anything in the world just to be slimmer. It's the feeling which has you saying, 'That's it! Starting right now, come hell or high water, I am no longer going to be fat, and I will do anything to make it happen!'

And many do just about *anything* to move away from fat. This can involve pills, starving themselves, 'slimming shakes', 'quick-fix' diets, shrink-wrapping themselves, surgery, jaw wiring – and even something as crazy as joining a gym and actually going, as well as buying fruits and vegetables and actually eating them!

Whatever you try, it will inevitably involve the use of tremendous amounts of willpower, discipline and control. It also usually involves going to bed early trying to 'sleep away cravings', missing many social gatherings 'in case you are tempted', and 'secret eating' of some kind. All of which adds up to the belief that getting slim is always hard and life is much more enjoyable when you are eating and drinking crap.

You continue with whatever method you are using to get rid of the excess fat until you reach a level *you* are comfortable with. Not a level of supreme health and a body of your dreams you understand; just where you are no longer as fat as you were and feel 'okay' with it. The second you reach that thought process the 'fat pressure' is released and **BOOM!** The downward slide begins *immediately*. As a 'reward' for all your hard work you inevitably 'treat' yourself. The 'treat', ironically, usually involves eating the same unsatisfying chemically loaded crap which made you start to hate yourself in the first place. You 'treat' and 'reward' yourself so much that before you know what has happened, you wake one morning, get a glimpse of yourself in the mirror and the involuntary thought, 'Oh shit! I'm fat again' rears its ugly head. The 'fat pressure level' has kicked in again and the same desperate cycle starts once more.

Taking it to Another Level

A Grand Design approach completely shatters this nightmare of a cycle. It changes the 'fat and health pressure' level and enables us to break the ceiling on what we deem the 'good enough level'. When someone is moving towards slim and healthy and not simply away from fat, the level at which they are happy is way beyond the Changing Diet ceiling of 'good enough'. When you focus on a Grand Design body and level of health, 'okay' and 'good enough' just don't cut it any more. You will find that when you hit what used to be your good enough level, you don't stop there and spiral back down. With a Grand Design approach you will find you move to a completely new level, a level of health and fitness you either have never experienced or experienced many years ago and have craved for so long. Grand Design is about creating a level of health and body shape that feels so good you will never want to leave – a place where you *love* to live.

Grand Design is about creating a level of health and body shape that feels so good you will never want to leave — a place where you LOVE to live.

Our body and mind are the only place we ever live. Yes, we may have a house, flat or whatever, and we may even choose to move away and live in different parts of the world. But the only place we ever really live is within our body and mind. This is why it doesn't matter how big someone's house is or how much money they have. If they are in a Changing Diets mentality and are suffering from FAT, they are in reality living in poverty.

if you don't look after your body you will have nowhere to live.

This is why having a Grand Design approach to your health from this point on is so important to your everyday living conditions. It is also of vital importance to your life expectancy. Let me be clear here: I don't mean how long you will actually live. No one can possibly ever predict such a thing, regardless of what you eat or drink or what mental attitude you have. I am talking about true life expectancy. It's about what you can expect to do today in your life. If the best you can expect for your life today is to get tired by late afternoon, numb yourself with chemical-laden 'food' and slump into your sofa watching television all night, then you have a very short life expectancy. If the best you can expect in your life today is just to 'get along' or 'put up with' or 'not be inspired to live your dream', then you have a very short life expectancy.

Juice Yourself Slim is about increasing life expectancy on every level. The 'juice' in the title is not simply about the drink. It's about getting that feeling back in your belly. It's about igniting that often elusive fire within, that spark which can make us want to build a true Grand Design body and mind. It's about feeling totally juiced as well as drinking it.

When you take your health and fitness to the next stage, your 'fat pressure' and 'good enough' levels change completely. You have effectively changed the settings on your fat and health thermostat. Even if/when you do 'dip' a little (we are all human, after all) that's all it will ever be – a little. You will have set a new standard for yourself, and you will always naturally adjust what you are doing slightly in order to make sure you get back to the level you now expect for yourself. *This* is the difference between being slim for a week and slim for life. *This* is the difference between Changing Diets and Grand Design.

Making the Build Effortless

On the television shows, a *Grand Designs* build always takes much longer than a *Changing Rooms* one. Anything worth building always takes time. Rome wasn't built in a day and all that. In the show, what often causes delays and stress for the owners is other people letting them down. The frustration is in not being in full control. However, whereas they have to rely on the skills of others, in this situation you are your own builder, surveyor, architect, project manager and interior designer all rolled into one. Even the build itself doesn't have to be stressful or take any massive degrees of effort, despite what we have been conditioned to believe.

It appears that everyone is under the false assumption that losing weight and getting healthy must always involve tremendous amounts of willpower, discipline, sacrifice and feelings of deprivation. In fact, this opinion is so ingrained that any suggestion that there is another way is always met with complete disbelief and instant dismissal. However, regardless of what is the accepted 'fact', the good news is there really is a way of thinking that makes the whole process of change not only easy but also enjoyable. It's a way of thinking that completely removes the need for willpower, discipline and control. It's a way of thinking which could, if adopted, radically change how people approach the whole process of changing what they eat, and would even be highly effective with other addictions too. There are usually two ways to go about any process of change. There is of course the difficult way, or indeed …

8

The Simple Way

The words simple, easy and enjoyable are not usually associated with losing weight, getting slim or embarking on any change of diet. But why not? Why shouldn't it be easy? We have accepted it's difficult to change our diet and get slim simply due to our own struggles or watching the struggles of others. But why should we all struggle? What exactly is so difficult about losing weight? What are we doing that is actually so hard? When you start to analyse it, it's not so clear. All we are doing is eating (or drinking in this case) a few different things to what we normally do, while cutting out a load of chemical-laden crap food from our diet and maybe starting a bit of exercise. What is so hard, seriously?

NASA: Never Accept Stereotypical Assumptions

When NASA was looking for a solution to the problem of writing in space, they looked no further than their own technology. After all, if NASA could put a man on the moon, coming up with a pen that could write in weightless conditions shouldn't have been much of a challenge. NASA spent 10 years and billions of dollars investing in new technology that would enable a pen to work at all times in zero gravity. The Russians, however, simply took a pencil!

This is a great story and one you may have heard. It isn't actually true – and it's one of those Chinese whisper fables that get talked about as fact. However, there was a company which did spend millions of dollars getting the 'zero gravity' pen off the ground (so to speak). These pens now sell for $50 each. I can't help thinking that spending millions of dollars producing a pen that works in weightless conditions when they only sell for $50 each and have such a small market wasn't the best move. Especially when many people simply save the 50 bucks and use a pencil!

This shows how common sense is sometimes much more important than scientific endeavour. The answer to the problem of being able to write in weightlessness was obvious … *but only once it was pointed out*. Exactly the same principle applies to getting slim and healthy. The collective opinion seems to be that losing weight is difficult, involves tremendous amounts of willpower, discipline and control and is a lifelong battle. The reality, however, is there is a simple way and, like the weightlessness pen/pencil, it become incredibly obvious when it's pointed out.

I am not saying people don't find it difficult to lose weight, because they do. Nobody would go through the nightmare of having their jaw wired or surgery if they thought it was simple. There also wouldn't be scientists all over the world trying to come up with an anti-fat pill that can make the process easy. However, just because most of the world believes it to be hard doesn't make it so.

It's like the Rubik's Cube of the 1980s. Most of the world believed, and still do, that it's an incredibly difficult puzzle to solve. This appears to be an accepted 'fact'. However, it is only because we tried and failed so many times and watched others trying and failing that we all become convinced that the puzzle was difficult. In other words, we have thousands of references to back up the 'fact' that the cube is hard. Exactly the same principle applies to weight loss and changing diet. We have all tried and failed so many times and watched tens of thousands (if not millions) of others all over the world struggling that we have God-knows-how-many references to back up the belief that it's very, very hard.

The reality is that both the cube and getting slim can be simple. With the cube, all you have to do is follow a simple set of instructions and anyone can do it – yes, anyone. With losing weight you simply have to switch your thinking *slightly* and anyone can find the process not only easy but enjoyable too.

The Problem is Mental – and so is the Solution!

The reason why people struggle when trying to change their diet and lifestyle comes down to one thing and one thing alone – a feeling of *mental deprivation*. Remove the feeling of mental deprivation and there is no struggle and the process becomes easy. That's it and that's all.

Think about it! When we change what we eat we automatically switch into 'deprivation mode' and immediately start to feel like we are missing out. But why? Why do we feel we are missing out? Why do we feel deprived? We have just stopped eating a load of crap that was making us fat and miserable and have started a process that will make us slim and healthy. We should, if we think about it, be feeling bloody excited and totally elated.

Yet everyone seems to begin any change of diet with a feeling of doom and gloom. We all effectively put ourselves into a mental tantrum, similar to a child being told they can't have something. Our collective theory appears to be that if we suffer the misery of this tantrum for long enough, time will solve our problem, the cravings will go away and we will reach the stage where we are totally happy about our new diet and fitness lifestyle.

With losing weight you simply have to switch your thinking SLIGHTLY and anyone can find the process not only easy but enjoyable too.

This may sound logical. However, as the cravings are *mental* and not *physical*, eventually you will give in and return to the foods and drinks you feel you are missing out on. The reason you give in is because you feel you have genuinely 'given up' something worth having. This leads to a feeling of sacrifice, and you start to feel mentally deprived. You start to envy people who are consuming the foods and drinks you have 'given up'. You start to feel hard done by and sorry for yourself. You feel your freedom of choice has been removed. Eventually the pressure builds and you start saying things like, 'Oh sod it! I could get run over by a bus tomorrow,' and before you know what's happened you are back on the crap again.

When you do go back on the crap, the mad thing is that it doesn't do what you convinced yourself it would. Yes, you may feel good initially but that's *only* because you have stopped your mental tantrum; its *not* because the crap actually makes you happier. You are happier simply because you are no longer feeling deprived, and no longer whining and moping around. In fact, it doesn't take long at all before you are once again saying, 'Oh shit! I wish I hadn't done that.' But once the seal is broken, everything goes pear-shaped, and you are usually on a downward spiral until your next 'I will change my life on Monday' declaration. It appears you are in a no-win situation. You are miserable when you do eat the crap and miserable when you don't!

However, there is a way out. We could always stop eating the crap, rejoice in our decision and feel excited about the fact that we will soon be slim and sexy! You may be thinking that if it was that easy everyone would do it, but why shouldn't it be that simple? From what I see, eating crap is not easy, and neither is eating it with a warped, deprived mind. As I've already mentioned, when you eat it you feel like crap, and when you don't eat it you feel miserable and deprived. But why should we feel down and deprived? Is it possible we have got the whole thing the wrong way around? I mean, what exactly are we being deprived of by stopping eating loads of crap and getting slim anyway? What exactly are we giving up?

Nothing to Give Up

This is the biggest irony of all. It is only when we *are* eating and drinking rubbish all the time that genuine deprivation occurs. We are being deprived of our health, our money, our peace of mind, our self-respect, our courage, our confidence and, of course, our freedom. The freedom to move the way we want; the freedom to wear the clothes we want; the freedom to be our natural selves, and the freedom to have genuine choice over what we eat. So often the choice has been made for us by clever, manipulative advertising and chemical-laden food designed to create additional *false* hungers. However, you cannot have genuine freedom of choice without the freedom to refuse. Let me repeat that:

You cannot have freedom of choice without the freedom to refuse.

Once you can refuse and be happy about it then, and only then, do you have true freedom of choice. When you are genuinely able to take or leave something, that's when freedom is yours. All the sacrifices are made when we are eating rubbish, not when we get rid of it. There is genuinely nothing to give up by making the change, and so much to give up by not making it. This is why it makes no sense to mope, whinge and drive ourselves mad when we stop overeating and/or consuming rubbish.

I said the struggle is all mental and this is perhaps the most mental part. When we stop doing the very thing we hated doing to ourselves we start moping because we are no longer doing it. Confused? Yes, it is confusing and slightly mad. It comes down to this: when we change what we eat we struggle because we effectively spend our time moping around for rubbish which we hope we won't have. Let me say that again:

We mope around for things which we hope we won't have.

How flipping mental is that – to feel deprived because you don't have something which you don't actually want! It is *only* the whingeing and moping that causes the problem. But what exactly are we pining for? What is so wonderful about empty foods that never truly satisfy on a mental or physical level, foods and drinks that make us fat, feel miserable and deplete our health insurance account? Seriously, what on earth are we really missing out on? Why on earth should we ever feel deprived, and if we see people putting cake after cake into their mouths, what on earth is there to envy? The madness is that when you start to *Juice Yourself Slim*, anyone who is eating crap all the time will be envying you! They would love to be in a Grand Design frame of mind. They would love not to be doing what they are. When they finish eating their crap, do they feel better than you? Have they actually gained anything, or do they feel like the very stuff they have eaten – crap?

When I was fat, unhealthy and consuming rubbish all the time, I would say and do anything to justify my actions. I would even accuse people who didn't join me of being boring and unsociable! But what is so boring about not eating crap, and how is someone being unsociable just because they aren't eating the same food as you? Are you ever boring and unsociable because you don't join them with eating an apple? Yes, that would be ridiculous, but no more so than the person who doesn't have a Death by Chocolate with their friends. They are still being sociable because they are out with their friends. The truth is those who do eat things like Death by Chocolate regularly will always need someone to 'join them' in the same way a smoker needs a fellow smoker to feel better about what they are doing.

Who is stopping you having anything you want? At any time during your *Juice Yourself Slim* life you can go to a shop and stuff your face – no one is stopping you. The choice at that stage is simple: either have whatever it is you are moping for and shut up or don't have it and shut up, but shut up! Sounds harsh, but it's *we* who are causing the problem by having this ridiculous mental tantrum. If we just stop moping around for things we hope we won't have, the tantrum is immediately removed and the process becomes simple and enjoyable.

And why shouldn't it be enjoyable? Why shouldn't we be excited? Why shouldn't we feel bloody elated? We are getting rid of the crap that was making us fat, miserable and ill and starting a lifestyle where we get to build our body and health Grand Design. A life where we can move freely and love the way we look, and a life where we know we are getting the best health insurance on earth. This is why most have got it wrong. They *start* with a feeling of doom and gloom and an attitude of 'getting through it'. They stop eating crap because they hated the way it made them feel, yet the second they stop and see other people eating this muck, they start to envy them! No wonder they fail.

Simple and Effective

All you need to do is:

- ✿ realize that there is nothing to give up
- ✿ make the concrete decision to build your Grand Design
- ✿ never ever question that decision
- ✿ never envy anyone eating rubbish
- ✿ rejoice in your new freedom
- ✿ get on with enjoying the build

If you follow these simple instructions, nothing can possibly stop you and you will love the process. Remember, no one is forcing you to *Juice Yourself Slim* – it's your choice. *You* are choosing not to eat crap all the time, and *you* are choosing to create a body where you want to live. People around you will be envying **YOU**.

You also have several advantages over those people who have never suffered from being overweight:

✿ **Very few people change what they eat unless they are overweight.**
   We are in an aesthetic world and looks, nine times out of ten, will win over health. Very few people change their diet to one of optimum nutrition unless they are overweight or ill. I see my psoriasis and tendency to gain weight just by looking at a cake as a blessing. There is no way I would consume the level of natural foods and drinks and exercise the way I do *unless* I was prone to overweight. There is no way I would enjoy my current level of

fitness and health unless I once suffered from these conditions. They were a massive incentive for me to do something about it. Naturally slim people don't have this same incentive. They often brag that they eat nothing but pizza, drink Coke, do no exercise and yet are thin as rakes. They say they are lucky because they 'get away with it'. The reality, however, is that they aren't getting away with it. Just because their body doesn't get fat doesn't mean it doesn't get sick inside. It is not a godsend to be able to eat whatever you like and not get fat. In fact, it can often be a curse. When you *Juice Yourself Slim* you will be slim, healthy and have an extremely strong health care system.

🌱 **You don't take your slim, healthy body for granted.** If a woman has been a size 10 or 12 all her life, or a bloke has always had a 32-inch waist and a six pack, they take it for granted. To them it's normal. However, if you have been a size 14/16/18/20 or have a 36/38/40-inch waist with a stomach that hangs *over* the belt, and all of a sudden you find yourself a size 10/12 or a 32-inch flat pack, you are going to be one happy camper. You will always have this reference when day-to-day problems occur. If something bad happens to you, you can always think, 'Yes, shit happens in life, but it could be worse. I could be fat!' Once you're free from the 'hook' to eat crap, it's wonderful when your brain automatically kicks in and says, 'It could be worse. I could have tried to "use" food to solve this problem, but thank God I'm free from having to do that.' If someone were to lose the use of their legs for a while and get that use back again, I can guarantee it would be a long time before they weren't ecstatic about being able to walk. Those who have always had this gift never get excited about walking, as they expect to be able to do it. When, like me, you have lived in a squat on the North Peckham Estate, anywhere else seems like a Madison Square penthouse!

🌱 **Personality!** Okay, this isn't 100 per cent accurate, but there is something in it. It has been said that many slim and gorgeous people have no personality. Now, clearly this can often come from rumours put out by a few, sometimes resentful and jealous, overweight people. However, sometimes it's true, and I believe this is for a very good reason. When you aren't the most attractive bunny in the field, your personality develops almost out of necessity. I was a little fat bloke covered from head to foot in psoriasis who used an asthma pump every half an hour – what a catch! Clearly, there was no way I could rely on aesthetics to meet people; I *had* to get a personality. Those 'stunners' can simply walk into a bar and they are instant magnets. They often don't have to say anything at all for people to want to be with them (sometimes it's best if they don't say anything). This is another great benefit to having once been overweight. When you *Juice Yourself Slim* you will be slim, trim *and* you will have a personality!

🍐 **As you shrink you grow!** This, I feel, is the biggest advantage. When we overcome any adversity in life we grow and expand our world. Like any *Grand Designs* project, at times there will naturally be challenges and things won't always be plain sailing. You should hope these times *do* come along. The vast majority of the time, juicing yourself slim will be pretty simple, but please cherish those times when you struggle either a little or a great deal. The growth is always in the struggle, so don't simply throw in the towel *when*, not *if*, these times occur. Find a way to overcome and relish them. When I see the people who build their Grand Design on television, I notice that when they overcome obstacles, their sense of achievement and appreciation is always greater. I know many people who simply want to fast-forward their lives. They say if there were a magic button they could press and be slim and trim one year on, they would press it. But the real juice is in the growth. By buying a ready meal and hiding the packets you may be able to convince your guests you cooked it, but you could never feel a sense of pride and achievement, and you won't have learnt anything to make you a better cook next time.

It's Called Self-help Because
You Have to Help Yourself!

By building your Grand Design and committing to do whatever it takes to make it happen, you will expand your life in more ways than I can possibly express here. The fat world and slim world are two very different places with extremely different atmospheric conditions. And the only way you will get from one world to the other is not by simply reading this book, but taking instant and massive action. Everything you have read in this book will mean jack without ACTION.

By buying a book of this nature you have done what a great section of the population does. By actually reading it you are way ahead of most. If you ACT upon the information you will enter an elite world of doers and not talkers. Anyone can talk about change, and that's what most people do – talk. They are always thinking about doing this or that, yet never seem to get around to anything other than the 'thinking about it' stage. The fact you have reached this page in this book means the huge chances are you are about to enter the world of 'doing' and not 'thinking'. You are tapping into the most valuable commodity we have: the ability to act.

I know loads of people who want to write a book but never put pen to paper. I know many people who say they want to lose weight but never put salad to plate! Whatever you are 'thinking' about doing in life, stop THINKING and just bloody do it! You feel sooooooooooooo good when you do and your spirit grows massively as a result. With that in mind, let's get on with it.

When you are physically BiG the world is a much smaller place.

Sink or Swim

There are usually two ways to go about something like this. You either take a gradual approach – which takes longer, is harder and is often followed by failure – or you can simply launch yourself into it.

It's like when you are at a swimming pool and the water is cooler than is comfortable. There are two ways in. You can gradually dip your toe in and climb down the steps very slowly or dive right in. If you choose the first option not only is the process slow and tortuous, you also run the risk of not swimming at all. If you choose the second option, the moment you are in you start swimming, and if it's uncomfortable at first, it feels bloody amazing once you get your momentum. The same applies here.

By now your mind should be itching to get started and that illusive fire within should have started to ignite. However, it is just as important to get your body firing on all cylinders as well as your mind. The huge chances are your body will be used to running on false stimulants like coffee, tea, sugar and so on, and many parts of your system will be toxic. In order for you to utilize the nutritional power within the juices, smoothies and live foods you eat, it is vital we have a clean-up first.

The first part of the *Juice Yourself Slim* lifestyle change is vital. You will not only lose about 7lbs during the first week – which will provide incredible momentum – but more importantly you will clear any 'false hungers'. This means that when you move on to the incredible, flexible, simple and almost foolproof Juice Yourself Slim *for Life* stage, your system and mind will be totally clear of any chemical-laden drug-like food influences. I cannot emphasize enough just how important the first part is on every level.

This book is all about igniting that fire within, and a touch of ignition is exactly what is required for this first part of *Juice Yourself Slim*. Before we enter the world where the whole thing becomes second nature – and to make sure we don't simply come crashing down – nothing is more important than …

9

The Launch

it takes 90 per cent of the space shuttle's energy to get it into space, but only 10 per cent to keep it there.

This is why I have devised the seven-day launch programme, and ask you not to deviate off course. The 'launch' will clean your system; you'll drop a good deal of weight; it will get rid of any 'withdrawal' from certain 'drug' foods; and will make you feel so good there is no way you won't want to continue.

What surprises most people is that they don't feel hungry during the launch. They see that it involves mainly juices, smoothies, soups and some salads. They assume they will be wanting to eat their own arm off by day three. However, because they were overfed and undernourished but are now getting good quality, 'live', easy-to-assimilate nutrition, they are, for once, genuinely being fed.

Feelings of Withdrawal

It is only during the first few days when you may at times feel a degree of excessive hunger. This will **NOT** be a genuine hunger but feelings of withdrawal. This withdrawal is a slight empty, insecure feeling which feels identical to normal hunger. When people stop smoking they tend to eat more food at first. This is because the empty, insecure feeling of nicotine withdrawal is very similar to a hunger for food. You will more than likely be 'withdrawing' from refined sugars, refined fats, artificial sweeteners, caffeine and so on. An automatic feeling may come into your head asking for a 'fix', which manifests itself as the words 'I'm hungry'. But please understand you are not genuinely hungry for any of that rubbish. These feelings, like any slight feelings of withdrawal, will soon go.

If the hunger continues or gets worse, this isn't anything physical. It is a mental hunger, simply a mental feeling of deprivation. You are in full control of this feeling and you can stop it any time you wish. Many people like these 'false hungers' and don't get anxious about them. In fact, they rejoice in being able to overcome them.

You may also find that as well as a few 'false hungers' here and there, you experience headaches and a loss of energy. The headaches are caused by the 'withdrawal' and will soon be gone. Just keep hydrated and **DON'T TAKE ANY HEADACHE PILLS** (unless you are on this medication already and have been told to take it daily by your GP). As for the energy loss, this is perfectly normal. Not everyone experiences it. Doing the exercises I recommend and feeling excited about the programme creates its own energy. However, some do get a slump. This is because it takes a few days for your body to learn how to tap into its own energy stores again. It is so used to being 'revved up' with sugars, caffeine, artificial sweeteners and the like that it has to 'learn' how to do it without them. This can take a few days and is another reason why the launch is so important. If you are sleeping more than usual during this week, allow yourself that luxury if at all possible.

Don't Force-Feed Yourself

Please don't worry if at any stage you don't have all of the juices, smoothies, soups and salads on a particular day. You may feel that won't happen to you, but I can promise you that when you start to feed yourself genuine nutrition which gets to the parts other foods cannot reach, you will be surprised at just how little food you actually require to thrive. If you really don't feel like a particular juice, smoothie or soup because you don't feel hungry – don't have it! Don't ever force food down yourself. Your body will know when it's hungry. Having said that, during this seven-day launch **DON'T EVER MiSS YOUR BREAKFAST JUiCE OR SMOOTHiE.** It is important to kick-start your metabolism in the morning.

We have been so conditioned to eat as a response to emotion or to what the clock says, we seemingly never eat as a response purely to a genuine hunger. Don't ever think 'I should eat' based on anything other than a genuine hunger. Sometimes I eat all day and other days I am not hungry at all. I eat when my body wants fuel, not when the clock says I should eat. If you ever get caught into a head space where you start thinking 'I have hardly had anything today, I really must eat', just ask yourself this one core question. This question alone can keep you slim for life:

'if i didn't know how much food i have had, how hungry would i really be?'

This principle is the same for many aspects of life. For example, if you didn't know how much sleep you had had, how tired would you really be? When in any doubt always ask, 'If I didn't know how much food I have actually had, how hungry would I really be?' Most of the time the hunger is mental, not physical at all.

Be Prepared!

Like any launch, preparation is the key to a successful mission. Without the right preparation, a sudden crash is likely. This is why I have provided the 'launch pack', in chapter 11. It lists everything you will need for a successful launch. It also contains a full shopping list and details of the programme itself. Make a point of reading it. One essential item is the launch wall planner; it really makes the programme much easier.

Reintroduce Other Foods and Drinks Gradually

During the seven day launch your body will grow to expect and enjoy the finest liquid fuel or live water-rich salads. Your body will also be free of white refined sugars, fats, man-made carbohydrates, dairy, meats, fish, chocolate, sweets, caffeine and alcohol. Your body will become a very efficient machine, and if you were to introduce all of the above on day eight you would understandably cause the body some degree of distress. After a detox programme of this nature some people can become 'blocked' if they nip off to the golden arches for a Big Mac, fries and coke.

After seven days on pure food your body will have become much more alkaline. You will notice that by the end of the launch, instead of wanting junk, you will find you are craving delicious healthy foods such as stir-fried veggies, lean meats, king prawns, brown rice, tuna, avocado and so on. Realistically, however, this is not always going to be the case. This is a programme for life and at times you will of course have other things. However, on the eighth, ninth and tenth days just use your head and reintroduce foods and drinks *gently*. In many cases you will find that you no longer 'need' to reach for your usual cup of double espresso to get you going in the morning; you will have broken the pattern and discovered at first hand the amazing natural high that a morning juice can generate.

You don't have to do the launch to *Juice Yourself Slim*. You can take a gradual approach by skipping it and simply adopting the core Juice Yourself Slim *for Life*. If you follow these easy core principles, you will naturally still achieve success. However, there is a chance – like the swimming pool analogy – of simply dipping your toe in and retreating. You have come this far in the book so why not take the plunge and just do the launch?

You may choose to do just three, four or five days of the launch and then go into the key Juice Yourself Slim *for Life* principles. Please remember the whole point of Juice Yourself Slim is to make life **EASY** and to enable you to get to, and *stay* in, the land of the slim and healthy effortlessly. If you follow the right way of thinking, even the launch will be a breeze and I would strongly recommend – especially in terms of laying the right health foundations and clearing your system – that you dive straight in and complete the launch in its entirety. The details of the launch are coming soon, but before you even start, it is vital you fully understand not just how to Juice Yourself Slim for seven days, but you fully understand everything you need to do in order to …

10

Juice Yourself Slim for Life

The Core Principles

The core principles of this lifestyle are perfect for anyone, whether you are juicing yourself slim *for life* or juicing yourself to amazing health and a solid natural health care system. This is why I particularly love *Juice Yourself Slim*. The core principles are short, precise and incredibly easy to follow, wherever you live and whatever your lifestyle. They are highly effective yet incredibly flexible. *Juice Yourself Slim* is a lifestyle. This isn't about simply juicing yourself slim and then going back to what made you fat to start with. This change is for life and is why these principles need to be as simple as possible to implement.

> JUiCE YOURSELF SLiM is a lifestyle. This isn't about simply juicing yourself slim and then going back to what made you fat to start with. This change is for life.

1. Replace two meals a day with a juice, smoothie or soup, five days a week.
2. Don't feed an emotion with food.
3. DO NOT OVEREAT!
4. Watch out for snacking!
5. Don't label it!
6. Eat your food and drink your juices slowly.
7. Move your body DAILY!
8. Keep your spirits high!
9. Use your culinary imagination.
10. The C.A.N.T. principle.

1. Replace Two Meals a Day with a Juice, Smoothie or Soup, Five Days a Week

This is the big one and the main principle behind juicing yourself slim *for life*. It may almost sound too simple, but it works!

Your new juicy lifestyle involves replacing two of your three regular meals with a juice, smoothie or soup, while your other meal can be whatever you desire. I am hoping by now that you love the juices, smoothies, soups and salads so much that you desire them. This is the pattern for five days of the week, then at the weekend you are free to be even more flexible. If you follow the same principle at weekends, the results are even more dramatic.

My aim is that by the time you get this far on the programme you will be truly free to choose foods that are good for you, and you will crave fewer empty foods which do nothing for you. The beauty of juicing yourself slim *for life* is its flexibility – that's why people like it and find it easy, and why it's something they can do for life. As long as you follow all the other principles, you can be incredibly free around food and still get the results you are looking for.

Many people choose to have a juice or smoothie for breakfast, a soup or smoothie for lunch and then a regular meal in the evening. The regular meal is often nutritious, such as a large salad, maybe a brown rice dish, some wholegrain pasta and pesto – you get the idea. Some prefer to go down the not-so-healthy meal route and tuck into fish and chips now and then.

The beauty of juicing yourself slim FOR LiFE is its flexibility — that's why people like it and find it easy, and why it's something they can do for life.

Others prefer to have a juice or smoothie for breakfast, eat a regular lunch and then have soup in the evening. At weekends, virtually all choose to have a juice in the morning and then maybe other stuff for the rest of the day – they are so used to getting their daily dose of health care they can't see why they need to change anything else. Others keep to the same principle as they have for the five days. Clearly it's your choice and depends on your lifestyle. If your family cherishes their evening meals together then it makes sense to enjoy the same meal, and have your liquid fuel for breakfast and lunch. If, however, you enjoy hitting the deli with friends or gastro pub with colleagues at lunchtime, your lifestyle is better suited to having your regular lunch and a juice or smoothie for breakfast and soup for supper. The choice is yours.

If you are very overweight then you will *Juice Yourself Slim* more quickly by sticking to the principle of juice/smoothie/meal (or whatever combination you have chosen) for as many days as possible. It is also clear that if you choose your meal to be fish and chips with half a loaf of bread every night, your journey to the land of the slim will be a much longer one.

Personally, I love to have a juice or smoothie in the morning. Often I simply have a juice for lunch and eat my main meal in the evening. At weekends I sometimes have just one juice a day, or occasionally none, depending on where I am. However, this may not work for you, so please do what works for *you*, not me! Whatever you do, though, don't bust a gut to juice at any cost. I know some people who take their juicer everywhere, even to a friend's house when staying the night. This is okay if you know them really well and they understand, but some-times it can come across as a bit strange and rude!

2. Don't Feed an Emotion with Food

If you are not genuinely physically hungry then anything you eat as a response to an emotion will turn to fat in the body. You simply can-not feed an emotion with food, and even good food will cease to be good if you are genuinely not hungry. Remember to always ask yourself the core question:

> 'if i didn't know how much food i had eaten,
> how hungry would i be?'

Never eat as a response to an emotion or indeed simply because the clock says it's dinner time and therefore you *must* be hungry. Learn to listen to your body and become an intuitive eater. We have been pro-grammed by **BiG FOOD** manufacturers to eat as a response to emotion, but part of any negative emotion was often caused by the last fix of **BiG FOOD** you had.

You may think you eat as a response to emotion but the fact is you eat *certain things* as a response to emotion. No one, to my knowledge, has ever said, 'I'm pissed off. I need a grape!' **BiG FOOD** creates **BiG EMO-TiONS** and fools us into thinking it can help. Don't fall for it. Life can often be challenging but if you are stressed you should look for the cause, and I can guarantee that the cause is never a Mars Bar defi-ciency! **ONLY EAT WHEN YOU ARE GENUiNELY HUNGRY.**

3. DO NOT OVEREAT!

If you want to *Juice Yourself Slim* and build your body and life to a Grand Design, keep to this principle. Just as it is important to eat only when you are genuinely hungry, it is essential to stop eating just before you are uncomfortably full. I realize this may take some training, but you are building your Grand Design here and this principle is core to laying the right foundations. There is no pleasure to overeating. You don't gain more pleasure from the food by having more of it. Once the body has had enough the sensation stops being one of pleasure and you feel bloated and stuffed. At times like Christmas you will inevitably forget this principle and experience, again, how awful it feels to be bloated. However, what you do most of the time determines your health and body shape – once in a while for anything won't interfere with your bigger picture.

4. Watch out for Snacking!

If you swap two meals a day for delicious, nutritious juices and smoothies then eat a salad for your evening meal you will see superb results in no time. However, if you do the above but also start munching on chocolate biscuits, blueberry muffins and crunchy Kettle Chips, your chances of success on this programme are slim.

If you really feel the need for a little something extra please see Chapter 12 (*page 160*) for some recommended snacks and things to eat 'on the move'. Clearly we all have different body types, jobs and physical and mental demands which all require different levels of energy. This is why it is important that you should eat if you are genuinely hungry. Just make sure it's something good. Also, keep in mind that the real pleasure in eating lies in the ending of a genuine hunger, so if you skip the unnecessary snacking, you will love your meals and juices all the more.

5. Don't Label it!

It is also important not to label yourself. The second you say, 'I'm a vegetarian/vegan/pescitarian' and so on you may be setting yourself up to feel deprived at some point. I am not saying don't be a vegetarian, vegan or whatever, just that there is no need for the label. Yes, you choose not to have animal produce but don't keep saying 'I'm a ...'. If it doesn't drive you nuts, it may have that effect on other people.

Talking of labels, I often get asked, 'What should I look to avoid on a label?' My answer is often **'THE LABEL!'** Natural foods don't have labels, although with increasing EU regulations, that might not be far away. I think if we all just ate **'NO LABEL'** foods 80 per cent of the time, all would be well. Think about it. Fresh fruits and vegetables, natural seeds and nuts and organic free-range meats and fish don't have labels. Obviously, when you go to concerts, football matches and the like there are many 'no label' foods for sale – I class these as 'mystery foods' as it's often a bloody mystery what's in them!

No, I am talking fresh produce with no labels – that's what you are really looking for. As for labels on food, I would skip anything you can't pronounce! That should sort the good from the bad. Okay, that's slightly too ambiguous, but I think you get my point. Watch out for things like 'organic' on anything other than fresh, no-label foods. I know many people who think 'organic' chocolate or sugar is good for them. Just because it's organic doesn't mean it's good for you. You can, after all, get 'organic cocaine' and 'organic heroin'! Also, don't be deceived by 'green' packaging and words like 'natural'. **BiG FOOD** and the government are often working together, and when you have a traffic light system apparently showing us what is good and bad, please don't assume they've got it right. Remember, their idea of pure natural health might be light years away from what your body actually needs. So in these cases, yes, check the label. Oh, and anything with trans-fats in it – **RUN A BLOODY MiLE!**

6. Eat Your Food and Drink Your Juices Slowly

This might seem like an off-the-cuff remark but it is really important, especially when it comes to your juices and smoothies. The digestion process starts in your mouth so take your time over sips. It takes a number of minutes for your brain to register that you have 'eaten' so if you gulp your smoothie down in five seconds, the chances are you will still feel hungry. How many times have you felt hungry after a meal and contemplated a dessert only to find 15–20 minutes later that the feeling has passed?

7. Move Your Body DAiLY!

It is so important to move your body as much as you can. Physical movement is a vital element of juicing yourself slim *for life* for many, many reasons. As well as helping with the slimming process, exercise makes the body firmer. You will also notice a decrease in your desire to eat crap; you will get an instant release of endorphins which will make you feel 'alive'; and you will probably start meeting a whole bunch of new people. You need to find a way of exercising that is fun so it feels like you are playing. Everyone will be different but maybe you would love to join a football or hockey club or start playing badminton with your partner, start jogging or get a mini-trampoline. Not all exercise needs to involve running or jumping about. In fact some of the finest exercise involves slow fluid movement. Yoga is perhaps one of the most excellent forms of exercise for body and mind. There are many yoga DVDs and classes out there. However, the guru of the discipline has got to be the Yoga Master himself, better known as Keith Ryan. His *Journey to Tranquillity* DVD is perhaps one of the best on the market. Clearly the type of exercise is up to you to decide. By moving your body on a consistent basis you will see major benefits, as well as a slim stomach. Remember: movement is life and no movement at all means you are dead!

8. Keep Your Spirits High!

Perhaps this is the most important principle. There are three things that enable us to live a longer life than most. Nutrition is not at the top of the list and neither is exercise. Spirit far exceeds anything else. I hope that after having read this book your inspirational juices are flowing. Nothing is more detrimental to health than losing that fire within. When our spirits are sky-high, it's no coincidence that our health usually follows. The chemicals released when we are excited about life are a whole different concoction to those we get when we are highly stressed. This is why it is vital to find as many ways to lift your spirits as possible.

Fill your life with things that excite you and keep the fire alive. Don't rely on one thing, as if that doesn't work out the way you expected, it is easy for your fire to die down. Every day you are on the journey of *Juice Yourself Slim* you have something exciting happening – you are building your Grand Design. However, once you are slim and the Grand Design is a reality, you will realize that life as a slim and fit person has its ups and downs. To avoid returning to 'fat land' it is important to find ways to keep that fire very much alive.

> **Fill your life with things that excite you and keep the fire alive.**

9. Use Your Culinary Imagination

This book contains some superb recipes which you can follow to the letter or just use as a guideline. You really need to enjoy what you are eating and drinking in order to feel fulfilled, so if you don't like a particular recipe simply skip it. Have some fun here and play around with your own combinations depending on what is in season or happens to be in your fridge.

However, it's important that you adhere to the basic principles of the recipes. For example, all the soups are made with no dairy, so if you start using full-fat milk, cheese and butter to make your soups you really have missed the point. Be creative with the juices as you really cannot go far wrong here, and the same goes for the smoothies unless you start using full-fat yoghurt and blended Mars Bars! I'm sure you get the idea and I expect that after your initial playing around you will find a few core recipes you love, and making them will soon become second nature to you. For further inspiration, you will find over 100 other recipes in my book *The Juice Master: Keeping it Simple*.

10. The C.A.N.T. Principle

If you feel your mind entering that 'I want but I can't have' mode, then **STOP!** Either change your thinking or have the food. This is a flexible lifestyle where you are completely free around *all* food and drink; where you can make the genuine and free choice to eat or drink whatever *you* want and not what others have manipulated you to 'choose' in the name of profit. Don't continue with any kind of self-imposed tantrum. Remember, it's *only* a feeling of mental deprivation that makes people believe it's hard to change their eating patterns – I cannot repeat this point enough.

Obviously, I am hoping that after you have read this book you will be much less likely to want as much of the empty crap, and that you will have a genuine desire for much of what you have been consuming during the launch. As I stated earlier, you **CAN** have whatever you like, but remind yourself why you wanted to cut down massively on the crap or get rid of it altogether in the first place. Then you automatically go from a 'I want but I *can't* have' **DIET** mentality to a much more liberating and totally free 'I *can* have it but I don't actually want to – I'm **FREE!**' In almost all my books on lifestyle change or addiction, I use – or remind people of – a good acronym to illustrate this point further:

C.A.N.T
Constant And Never-ending Tantrum

If you simply remove the 'T' and understand that at any given time you can have what you like, the 'tantrum' is immediately removed. This is the difference between a 'diet mentality' and one of 'food freedom'.

For *Juice Yourself Slim* to be effective it is imperative that you are free around food. And by 'effective' I don't simply mean you getting slim. I mean a total sense of freedom around all food and drink. This means you are free to have them if you want to. The only question you should ask most of the time is, 'Why on earth would I want to?' It is also good, if you do feel you are about to eat a load of crap, to ask, 'What would it genuinely do for me?' If you are doing it out of emotion, ask yourself how on earth this 'food' could possibly feed any emotion. If you are doing it out of a genuine hunger then ask yourself, 'Will this "food" genuinely satisfy me or simply leave me feeling empty in no time at all?'

Final Thoughts

Please remember that most of the so-called food industry has no intention of supplying food that will genuinely satisfy your nutritional and fuel requirements. **BiG FOOD** is **BiG BUSiNESS** and the only way to sell you more food is to either:

- ❧ Chemically change it so it doesn't genuinely satisfy, or
- ❧ Convince you through clever manipulative advertising that their food can change the way you feel.

What usually happens is a combination of the two. Food manufacturers are very clever with how they trap you and convince even the most rational thinker that a chocolate bar can cheer them up. The real pleasure in eating food is the ending of a hunger. Hunger is an empty, insecure feeling. When we eat food we stop this feeling and so feel good. The bigger the feeling of hunger, the more we relish the food. What we are actually enjoying is the ending of an aggravation. When we end any aggravation it feels good. If, for example, you have been skiing or snowboarding all day, the feeling you get when you eventually take off those boots is one of sheer bliss, almost euphoria. However, it's not a real pleasure. All we have done is end a large aggravation. The longer we have the boots on, the *more* pleasure we get when we remove them.

This same principle applies to **BiG FOOD**. Manufacturers produce 'food' which often causes blood sugar levels to drop lower than if you had eaten, say, an apple. On top of this they are also 'nutritionally short', meaning your body isn't being properly fed. This means they have created a way for you to feel hungrier than you normally would.

As the **real pleasure we get from eating is created by the ending of the aggravation of hunger**, they have very cleverly managed to delude us that their 'foods' give us more pleasure. This is why so many people feel a sense of sacrifice when they make a decision to stop eating them.

The irony is that there is no genuine pleasure to 'give up'. All that the **BiG FOOD** manufacturers have done is made us feel stronger levels of hunger more often. Therefore, every time we 'top up' with another 'fix' we feel a greater degree of pleasure than if we ate an apple. But it's a trick – and an ingenious one at that. Perhaps that's why one of the Mars Bar advertising slogans was 'pleasure you can't measure'. One of the genuine pleasures you get when you stop being a slave to these foods is to say **'UP YOURS!'** to **BiG FOOD**, and rejoice in the fact you are no longer part of their game and helping to fund their often unscrupulous enterprises.

That's it and that's All

Yes, those are the principles and that's all there is to it – hardly rocket science. Some people will be asking, 'But what can I have for the meal?' and would like a set meal plan to work from. However, this would mean there is no flexibility or freedom, and that would defeat the beauty of *Juice Yourself Slim*.

Many will ask 'Where are the rest of the recipes?' But the idea is to give control to you. There are more than enough good recipe books out there with gorgeous foods. Remember – you didn't misread – you can have **ANYTHING** for the one main meal a day. For best results, have something healthy, but at times you may choose something else. As long as you eat only when genuinely physically hungry, chew thoroughly and stop just before you are full, you will *Juice Yourself Slim* almost regardless of what you choose as your main meal and whatever you have at weekends. Clearly, if you are having 10 pints of beer a night then this isn't going to work. But then if you are, it's not so much juice you need as a different kind of help!

You now have all the mental and physical tools required to *Juice Yourself Slim*. There are over 60 recipes in this book and I have provided some nutritional facts about every single one. That way it gives you even more reason to start juicing yourself slim *for life*.

I would strongly advise reading the 'Questions 'n' Answers' section *in full (see page 273)*. What will also be of incredible value is the 'Juice Yourself Slim *on the move*' chapter *(see page 160)*. It's only a few pages and will tell you the best things to eat and drink when you are out and about. In fact, as mentioned at the start of this book, every word is written for a reason, so please don't make the mistake of missing theses sections.

I think I have covered everything and done all I can my end. It's up to you now. I would **HiGHLY** recommend starting your new or rejuvenated juicy lifestyle with the seven day launch programme before moving onto the incredibly flexible Juice Yourself Slim *for life* lifestyle. It will clean your body, enable you to drop shedloads of weight and reignite your fire in super-fast time. Your cravings, if any, will be fully eliminated, you will feel light and bright, and you'll have the slimmer's most sought-after commodity – momentum. All you need for launching into a healthier lifestyle is coming next.

At this point I would like to thank you for taking the time to read this book and persevering through the constant repetition which, as I explained earlier, is there for a good reason. I would love to hear your story. The more letters and emails we get, the stronger our argument for getting juice therapy recognized as a treatment and preventative for disease, especially the disease of being overweight. Your letters not only help this cause but are also, I believe, the biggest catalyst for change for others. When you read people's genuine testimonials, you are inspired beyond belief to juice yourself to health. I will leave you with a few more to help keep that fire alive, that fire that life sometimes dulls but is nevertheless ever present. Every now and then you simply need something to boost the flames. I hope this book has done just that. Once again, the following letters are 100 per cent genuine and come from people who have literally juiced themselves slim.

So unless I see you on a retreat or at a seminar, and in case I don't ever get to meet you personally, I sincerely wish you and those close to you a disease-free and enjoyable life. Remember:

Unless you look after your body you will have nowhere to live, and the only place you ever truly live is within your body.

'Thank you, Jason Vale. it took me five weeks on a different diet before the summer to achieve the same weight loss (8lbs in eight days) and i definitely didn't feel this good. i have started to make the juices for my children. They love them and i can't think of an easier way to get the same quantity of vitamins and minerals into them. They definitely wouldn't eat spinach and celery, etc.

Anyway, i'm glad i happened upon your book on Amazon — pure stroke of luck.

Kathy'

'Hi there
i must thank Jason for the fantastic book he's written and for giving me the inspiration to 'get juicing'. Carrying out this programme has given me back the confidence i had lost after going on many diets.

Thank you, thank you, thank you! Great book, easy-to-follow programme and i am 28lbs lighter as a result.

Debbie'

‘ i have lost 8lbs in just the first seven days of the JUiCE YOURSELF SLiM programme. i know i will have no problem with continuing the programme. The juices are gorgeous, the soups divine and i am not struggling one little bit as i have done before when trying to lose weight. Thank you for your inspiration.

Anna ’

‘ Hi there
i just wanted to say that i am on day four now and have never felt better! i didn't expect to feel this good. What amazes me is that i seem to have broken through my psychological barrier of eating at the slightest sign of (what i thought was) hunger. it is also so much easier to follow than other programmes. i find myself looking forward to the juices. i am sure you get lots of feedback like this but i just wanted to let you know how life-changing this experience is proving to me!

Many thanks
Natalia ’

11

The Launch Pack

As I have mentioned, before embarking on any great voyage or journey it is important that you do the right preparation to ensure a smooth liftoff. During your initial launch to *Juice Yourself Slim* for life it is imperative that you maintain your momentum for the entire seven days by having the right support in place. With this in mind, you are going to need the following:

Essential Equipment

I have made sure that at juicemaster.com we have everything for people's juicy needs in a one-stop shop. However, some people think this isn't for your convenience but for my profit. With that in mind, you can get everything you need in shops on the high street, but you can't get it all in just one shop, which is genuinely why I have the site.

Juice Extractor

It shouldn't come as a surprise that in order to *Juice Yourself Slim*, you will need a juicer. When I say a juicer, what I mean is the *right* juicer. There is nothing like an old style, 'dial-up internet connection' juicer to put your juicing life into an early grave! In order to *Juice Yourself Slim* for life *easily*, you may also decide to invest in a second machine for your place of work.

Today we are in an age of 'broadband' juicing, where a machine can easily take three whole apples and produce the finest apple juice with no peeling, coring or chopping. For the past two years I have been recommending the Philips aluminium wide-funnel juicer, and to this day I still believe 100 per cent that this is the best domestic juicer in its category on the market. The latest one is the HR1861 but they upgrade all the time. I have tested many, many juice extractors and I am still blown away by the supremacy of this machine. It extracts as much as 70 per cent more juice than some conventional juicers; it looks about as slick as it gets; it 'purrs' when you use it; it has a wide funnel and a separate pulp container and is dishwasher friendly.

> **Today we are in an age of 'broadband' juicing, where a machine can easily take three whole apples and produce the finest apple juice with no peeling, coring or chopping.**

It's not just me who sings this machine's virtues from the rooftops. It has been voted a 'Best Buy' by *Which?* magazine, and 'Best Juicer' in *Good Housekeeping* magazine for the last two years running. It scored 10 out of 10 in the *Daily Mirror* when pitched against many other juicers, and was voted 'Best Value' by *First* magazine. As I write it is the best-selling juice extractor in the UK, Ireland, Denmark, Sweden, Finland, Norway, Turkey, Italy, Germany, Holland and many other countries around the world – that's quite an impressive résumé by anyone's standard! Plus, at the time of this writing, you get a **FREE** copy of my best-selling glossy recipe book *Keeping It Simple* inside, no matter where you buy it.

If you own a masticating juicer, you can use it for the whole programme. Masticating juicers are excellent machines, but they can be expensive and take a lot longer to make a juice. They tend to extract more juice and the quality of the juice is excellent. The best ones on the market at the time of writing are The Champion, Green Star and

Madstone. The Champion was designed for fruit as well as veggies, whereas machines like the Green Star, which has a magnetic twin gear system, are mainly designed for veggies and struggle with watery fruits. The only thing a Champion won't do is wheatgrass, whereas the excellent Green Star and Madstone do. However, all masticators take much longer to make a juice so if time is of the essence, skip this type of juicer. Read more about all types of juicers at www.juicemaster.com to make an informed decision.

If you have an old juicer in your cupboard, please feel free to dust it off and crack on – any juicer will do. But, I will repeat, this is an investment for life. The right tools can make the difference between juicy success and juicy 'pain in the arse', followed by failure. If you are going to do it, do it right!

Technology is constantly improving and there will be many more advancements when it comes to juicing machines. So, depending on when you read this book, my recommendations may have been superseded, so please double check our website for the latest information.

Blender or Smoothie Maker

A blender and a smoothie maker are one and the same thing. There are many excellent blenders on the market and some pretty poor ones. When choosing a blender make sure it can blend ice and frozen fruit effortlessly. Philips do a blender which matches their juicer, so if reliability and aesthetics are important to you then look no further. If you feel you want something more powerful, then perhaps the best blender on the market today is the Vitamix, but they're about £500!

Hand Blender

To blend the soups you can either use your regular blender or invest in a hand blender. You really don't need both, but if you have a hand blender as well then you can simply blend the soup in the pan and only need to wash up the small attachment.

Flask

This is necessary for when you need to make your juices, smoothies or soups in advance for the day ahead. See our recommendations at juice-master.com.

Optional Extras

- **Wall planner.** We have developed a handy *Juice Yourself Slim* wall planner that you can stick on your fridge. The wall planner outlines all the recipes and how to make them, and gives you a day-by-day list of which recipes to have when. This is only available on our website, in Tesco NutriCentres and in our Juice Master Juice Bars; it only costs a few pounds. You can, of course, do the launch without it, but it makes it so, so much easier than having to refer to the book all the time.

- **Juice Master's Ultimate Superfood or Ultimate Juice Booster**. These powders are important for times when you cannot juice as they can simply be mixed with water to top up your health bank account. They also add extra nutrition when organic produce isn't being used.

- **Wheatgrass powder.** This can be added to some of the smoothie recipes and is to be found in all good health stores or on our website. You can also juice fresh wheatgrass but you need a separate wheatgrass juicer or masticating juicer. There are few things on this planet that are as powerful in terms of health as pure wheatgrass juice or good-quality powder. Go to Google and read up on the stuff; it's ridiculously good.

- **Juice Master's Variety Pack**. This contains a 50g bottle of Berry Boost, Clear Skin Boost, Ultimate Juice Boost, Ultimate Detox Boost and Love Boost. These boosters can be added to juices and smoothies during the seven-day launch and beyond.

- **Mini-trampoline.** Not all rebounders are built the same, what you are looking for is one with a 'soft' bounce. Most machines on the market have a very 'hard' and jarring bounce. These can often defeat the object of a good rebounder as they were designed not to jar the joints. See juicemaster.com for recommendations.

- ♀ **Yoga mat, trainers, swimsuit, skipping rope ...** Essentially anything that will get you moving. Exercise is SO important and I rely on a variety of activities to keep me inspired and motivated and, most importantly, to ensure I enjoy working out. We all need variety in our lives, especially when it comes to exercise. It's so easy to get bored, so mix it up. One day hit the gym, the next go for a one-hour walk or have a 20-minute skipping session – you get the point. Just find something you enjoy and you won't even realize you're working out.

- ♀ **MP3 or MP4 player.** As far as I am concerned this is a must. I realize this item may be expensive but there are many makes on the market other than the famous iPod, which all do pretty much the same job. In case this technology is new to you, an MP3 player is effectively a music player, and an MP4 player plays films too. Music is such an amazing stimulant for exercise. I love to run, but running to music is in a different world (unless I'm running on a beach!). Running is the same exercise over and over again, but one element I can always change is the music. Many times a certain tune kicks in and **BOOM!** An extra spark of energy is suddenly there. An MP4 player can be even better. Sometimes exercising on a stationary bike, for example, can be boring after a while. However, with an MP4 player you can download movies, sitcoms, documentaries and so on, and watch as you exercise. Before you know where you are, you've exercised your way through an entire film (but maybe not *Titanic*, which is three hours too long!). Personally, I like anything with Ricky Gervais – the man is a comedy genius. You could even download some juicy motivational stuff from our website to keep you inspired, helpful – especially during the first week.

Shopping List for the Seven-day Launch

You can also download this list free from juicemaster.com

Until recently, new out-of-town supermarkets and supermarket 'local' stores seemed to be popping up every five minutes. Local shops were in danger of dying a slow death. Luckily, change is happening. Increasing numbers of people are searching out farmers' markets, locally grown produce and organic delivery boxes.

In my old haunt of East Dulwich, southeast London, old-style shops are opening all the time. There's an organic butcher, an organic fruit and veg shop, an organic fishmonger and even a healthy fish and chip shop! Yes, you can go in and get fresh tuna and monkfish to have with your organic potato chunky chips. This is all happening a stone's throw from a massive Sainsbury's. Both supermarket and local shops are thriving and living side by side in a degree of harmony. I hope this will happen more frequently as people become increasingly aware of how their food is produced. Many supermarkets now also supply a good range of organic produce, but if the farmers' market comes to town, support it.

What You Will Need for the Next Seven Days

❧	Apples	x 28 (Golden Delicious are best; Granny Smiths are just wrong)
❧	Pineapples	x 5 (medium)
❧	Pears	x 2
❧	Courgettes	x 3
❧	Avocados	x 6 (organic if possible)
❧	Carrots	x 15 (small to medium)
❧	Parsnips	x 2 (medium)
❧	Cucumbers	x 5
❧	Beetroots	x 2 (raw NOT cooked)
❧	Celery	x 1 bunch
❧	Spinach	x 1 large bag of baby leaf
❧	Watercress	x 1 bag

❦ Mixed salad leaves	x 1 bag (100g)	
❦ Watercress, spinach & rocket	x 2 bags (140g bags)	
❦ Red pepper	x 1	
❦ Yellow pepper	x 2	
❦ Fennel	x 1 bulb	
❦ Lemons	x 3	
❦ Limes	x 4	
❦ Ginger	x 1 very small claw	
❦ Alfalfa sprouts	x 50g	
❦ Leeks	x 2	
❦ Broccoli	x 1 head	
❦ Butternut squash	x 1	
❦ Sweet potatoes	x 4 (medium)	
❦ Cherry tomatoes	x 12 (stalks removed)	
❦ Sun-blushed tomatoes	x 100g	
❦ Spring onions	x 1 bunch	
❦ Red onions	x 4 (small)	
❦ Garlic	x 2 cloves	
❦ Red chilli	x 1 (small)	
❦ Banana	x 1	
❦ Mixed berries	x 150g of fresh or frozen	
❦ Bio-live yoghurt	x 1 (450g) tub	
❦ Muesli	x 1 small bag	
❦ Olive oil	x 1 small bottle	
❦ Balsamic vinegar	x 1 small bottle	
❦ Good-quality vegetable stock cubes	x 7	
❦ Pepper	for seasoning the soups	
❦ Pesto	x 100g jar	
❦ Half-fat coconut milk	x 1 can	
❦ Spirulina*	x 1 small bottle (50g max)	
❦ Fresh mint for tea and some herbal teas		

* Spirulina can be found in all good health-food stores or on juicemaster.com

✿ Ice cubes

Clearly you can make these but ensure you have plenty made up ready.

The Launch Programme

Welcome to 'the launch'. The programme itself is extremely straight-forward. All the juices, smoothies, soups and salads have been carefully thought through to give you maximum benefits during the first seven days. What isn't listed is **exercise**. I have already mentioned just how important physical movement is to your mental and physical health. The minimum I would advise is two 20-minute exercise sessions daily, ideally first thing in the morning and before your evening meal. However, as a launch requires more energy than any other part of the mission, I would advise doing much more than that. You may not think you have the time, but the same people who say that seem to know what's happening in a few soap operas and the latest reality television show. Exercise is vital to the launch so get moving!

Recipes for all the juices, smoothies, soups and salads listed here can be found later in the book. I've used the term 'Linner' for the meal that comes between lunch and dinner!

KEY
Sm = smoothie
J = juice
Sp = soup
Sd = salad

Monday (or Day 1)

On waking   Hot water and lemon or fresh mint
Breakfast   Organic Avocado Crush (*Sm*) – pages 206–7

Brunch	Beta-Carrot Juice (*J*) – page 173
Lunch	Fennel Fuel (*Sm*) – page 215
'Linner'	Sweet Veggie Heaven (*J*) – pages 188–9
Dinner	Butternut Squash and Carrot Soup (*Sp*) – pages 232–3

Tuesday (or Day 2)

On waking	Hot water and lemon or fresh mint
Breakfast	Blood Builder (*Sm*) – page 212
Brunch	Sweet 'n' Savoury (*J*) – page 179
Lunch	Spirulina Smoothie (*Sm*) – pages 222–3
'Linner'	Body Balancer (*J*) – page 181
Dinner	'Souper' Green Stuff (*Sp*) – pages 234–5

Wednesday (or Day 3)

On waking	Hot water and lemon or fresh mint
Breakfast	Super Sporty Fuel Smoothie (*Sm*) – pages 218–19
Brunch	Sweet Veggie Heaven (*J*) – pages 188–9
Lunch	Bio-live Berries (*Sm*) – page 221
'Linner'	Body Balancer (*J*) – page 181
Dinner	Hunky Chunky Vegetable Soup (*Sp*) – pages 238–9

Thursday (or Day 4)

On waking	Hot water and lemon or fresh mint
Breakfast	Fruity Bio-live Breakfast Smoothie (*Sm*) – pages 216–17
Brunch	Spinach Stout (*J*) – page 183
Lunch	Fennel Fuel (*Sm*) – page 215
'Linner'	Sweet 'n' Savoury (*J*) – page 179
Dinner	Spinach, Watercress, Rocket and Sweet Potato Soup (*Sp*) – pages 250–1

Friday (or Day 5)

On waking	Hot water and lemon or fresh mint
Breakfast	Blood Builder (*Sm*) – page 212
Brunch	Beta-Carrot Juice (*J*) – page 173
Lunch	Super Sporty Fuel Smoothie (*Sm*) – pages 218–19
'Linner'	Spinach Stout (*J*) – page 183
Dinner	Sweet Cherry Tomato and Roasted Pepper Soup (*Sp*) – pages 246–7

Saturday (or Day 6)

On waking	Hot water and lemon or fresh mint
Breakfast	Bio-live Berries (*Sm*) – page 221
Brunch	Sweet Veggie Heaven (*J*) – pages 188–9
Lunch	Sweet Potato, Coconut and Chilli Soup (*Sp*) – pages 240–1
'Linner'	Organic Avocado Crush (*Sm*) – pages 206–7
Dinner	Green Pesto Power Salad (*Sd*) – page 253

Sunday (or Day 7)

On waking	Hot water and lemon or fresh mint
Breakfast	Fruity Bio-live Breakfast Smoothie (*Sm*) – pages 216–17
Brunch	Spinach Stout (*J*) – page 183
Lunch	Pear and Parsnip Soup (*Sp*) – pages 242–3
'Linner'	Spirulina Smoothie (*Sm*) – pages 222–3
Dinner	Avocado, Alfalfa and Sun-blushed Tomato Salad (*Sd*) – pages 266–7

12

Juice Yourself Slim on the Move

When juicing yourself slim there will inevitably be times when you are on the move and need some good-quality nutrition you can carry around. Luckily, contrary to what many people think, eating or drinking healthily when out and about is extremely easy. Here are a few suggestions.

Fresh Organic Fruit – the Perfect Food on the Move

When you are out, remember that you are always carrying an in-built juice extractor and blender with you. Your mouth is your blender and your digestive system is effectively one big juicer, and they work incredibly well when dealing with fresh fruit. Our systems were primarily designed with fresh organic fruit in mind, and nothing could be more perfect as a snack to eat on the move.

Your mouth is your blender and your digestive system is effectively one big juicer, and they work incredibly well when dealing with fresh fruit.

Fruit is incredibly easy to digest and packed with nutrients. Despite the average fruit containing over 80 per cent juice (even bananas), it comes in a solid form which makes it easy to carry. Organic fresh fruit is also 100 per cent degradable, which is good to know if you are worried about the planet.

So next time you feel the 'need' for a snack, don't forget the satisfaction that can be derived from a bag of juicy ripe cherries, a bunch of chilled grapes, a ripe juicy nectarine or a bowl of rich blueberries, summer strawberries and delicate raspberries.

Juice 'n' Go

If you really don't want to be without your juice, there are two ways you can easily stay juiced when out and about. First, you can always make enough juice in the morning to last throughout the day. This is particularly helpful as there will no doubt be times when you want to take a juice or smoothie somewhere to have later. Simply make some juices or smoothies in the morning and store them in the fridge in an air-tight flask.

It is important that you use the right kind of flask. If you're having problems finding a suitable one, please contact juicemaster.com. We have teamed up with the world-famous Swiss flask company, Sigg, who make the perfect lightweight juicing flask. The flask must be dark so that light cannot penetrate it. You should fill the flask right to the top – ideally, even allow a little of the drink to spill out as you secure the top to ensure there is absolutely no air in the flask. These two points are really important as light and air start the oxidation process and will greatly reduce the shelf life of your drink. If you keep your juice or smoothie in a dark, airtight flask in the fridge, it will be perfectly good for at least 12 hours.

As soon as you make a juice or smoothie its enzyme activity starts to decrease. Indeed, any juicing author worth their juicy title will tell you that for maximum health benefits the drink should be consumed as soon after it is made as possible. As the hours tick by, the mineral and vitamin content – as well as vital enzyme activity – will slowly degenerate. However, the science and juicing community have no conclusive evidence as to exactly how long a juice will retain enzyme activity after it is made. Even two or three days after being made a juice is still worth drinking in terms of its nutritional value. It certainly might not taste as good but it will arguably still have more health benefits than most pasteurized juices, and still be in a different league to a can of sugar-laden coke or other so-called 'soft' drinks.

Fresh Juice Bars

A second way to stay juiced when out and about is to find a *true and genuine* juice bar. This can be more difficult than you might think. I feel passionately about this as many 'juice bars' simply masquerade as the real thing while selling sugar-laden smoothies made from concentrated or pasteurized juice.

Another massive misconception is when a juice bar promotes its smoothies as 'made with fat-free yoghurt' but on closer inspection you discover this is made with up to 40 per cent sugar, not to mention an assortment of flavours and additives. Please remember: if you eat refined sugar and the body doesn't require it for energy it gets stored in **FAT CELLS**. This makes a complete mockery of most 'fat-free' claims. Many consumers believe they are getting a healthy smoothie when, in fact, they could be getting more calories than are found in a burger – at least with Burger King you know where you are! So keep vigilant and only buy juices and smoothies from genuine companies that actually juice the produce in front of you.

Some bars may only offer fresh apple, carrot or orange juice, which is still better than most. If you ask them to blend some fresh apple juice with a banana and some frozen berries you can get a fresh, great tasting, healthy smoothie at almost any juice bar. The smaller, individual juice bars are usually genuine and offer ingredients such as fresh spinach, pineapple, ginger, celery, cucumber, lemon and beetroot.

Out of my frustration, I decided to open my own Juice Master Juice 'n' Smoothie Bars to offer people *pure* fruit and vegetable juices and smoothies, and to be in a position to highlight the deceptions amongst many juice bars.

Just Add Water

If you genuinely cannot juice or prepare one in advance then there's an alternative that's particularly useful when you're out of produce, on a plane or on holiday. 'Power greens' is a generic term I apply to several different brands of powdered green vegetables, grasses, algae, friendly bacteria and so on. These are far from just vitamin or mineral substitutes; these powders offer an array of natural fruits, vegetables and plants that we would find it virtually impossible to find, let alone consume, on a daily basis. For this reason it's also worth taking 'power greens' a few days a week in conjunction with juicing as they contain superfood vegetation such as wheatgrass, spirulina, alfalfa, flax seed, enzymes, probiotics, echinacea and many other types of vegetation that we would never normally consume or juice.

These powders work just like the plant life in any desert. They can lie dormant beneath the surface for months on end and then, as soon as the life force that is water is applied, **BOOM!** They spring to life and in no time at all a sparse desert can be transformed into an oasis of vegetation. The vegetation in these powders is harvested and dried at very low temperatures so that its life force has essentially been paused. As soon as water is applied, it is like resurrecting the vegetation so that it springs back to life and has as many health benefits as the day it was harvested.

There are a few different varieties of 'power greens' available, not all of which are as pure as they might first appear, and many contain cheap fillers. I have also had difficulty finding a brand that dissolves completely in water and doesn't leave a bitty consistency. For me this is really important because 'power greens' are not only superb for adding to your juices or smoothies but are also a real emergency fall-back that can be mixed with water or shop-bought cloudy apple juice when you cannot juice. For this reason I developed my own blend of superb boosters and supplements which contain 100 per cent pure ingredients and 0 per cent fillers. What's more, all the ingredients are pulverized into a fine powder, which means they mix completely with water. To see the full range please visit juicemaster.com or check out a Juice Master juice bar and take a look at the 'Ultimate Juice Boost' and 'Ultimate Superfood'. I would also recommend Dr Udo's 'Beyond Greens' and Dr Robert Young's 'Inner Light Super Greens' as these, too, are good, genuine products.

Energy Bars

I do realize that we are all human and sometimes fresh fruit or juice is simply not going to cut the mustard. Personally, I like to grab one of those 'energy bar' type things when out and about. However, as with every aspect of the food world, it appears profit comes way ahead of genuine nutrition. Once again, words such as 'natural' and 'healthy' are plastered all over 'green' packaging, giving the often false impression we are getting a perfectly healthy 'energy' bar. Watch out for bars loaded with sugar, refined fats or artificial sweeteners. Even when most of the ingredients are perfectly good, you don't always get value for money.

Due, once again, to my frustration at the poor quality or rip-off 'energy bars' on the market today, I have developed my own. The Juice Master's **PURE ENERGY** *on the go* and **PURE JUICE IN A BAR** ranges can be found in many leading stores, supermarkets and juice bars and at juicemaster.com. They contain things like wheatgrass juice, parsley juice, broccoli juice, alfalfa and spinach, all of which would not win any awards on the taste front, but combined with apple juice powder and some other fine fruits, they taste gorgeous. They aren't the cheapest, but my philosophy is you get what you pay for, and when it comes to fuel for your body and your health insurance, it's the one area where we really don't want to compromise. Other good bars on the market include Nakd and The Food Doctor range.

13

Super Boost Me!

The subject of using any kind of nutritional supplement has always been a tricky one for me. After all, the main ethos behind juicing is to use the very best nature has to offer in the form that's easiest to absorb. Because you won't find a vitamin or mineral pill tree anywhere in nature, I never saw the need for any kind of vitamin or mineral supplements.

However, our overpopulated, commercialized 21st-century lifestyle has changed my view slightly. I still maintain that fruits and vegetables, and their organic juices in particular, are without doubt the best source of vitamins and minerals on earth, but now I do see there are certain times when a ' nutritional boost' can be extremely beneficial.

As I mentioned earlier, intensive farming has massively depleted our arable soils of vital minerals, so produce grown in such soils is low in certain minerals such as selenium and zinc. Please understand this is just what we know about. There are no doubt hundreds of nutritional co-factors missing too; we just can't pinpoint them at this stage. (Co-factors are 'helper molecules' that assist in the body's biochemical processes.)

The inferior nutritional content of such produce is then compounded by the application of pesticides, fungicides and chemical fertilizers, which furnish our fruits and vegetables with a dishonourable chemical concoction. Add to this a selection of genetically modified and chemically ripened produce and you have a bespoke harvest of not-so-desirable produce for the multimillion-pound fruit and vegetable industry. Contrast this to the 'earthy' produce that can be found at your local farmers' market, in your own back garden or in your organic veggie box, and you get a hunch that aesthetics and flavours have been distorted and the nutritional content may have been greatly compromised too.

it has been reported that you would need to eat an average of five apples today to get the same nutritional content as you would have found in just one apple 50 years ago.

As mentioned earlier, it has been reported that you would need to eat an average of five apples today to get the same nutritional content as you would have found in just one apple 50 years ago. It is because of this nutritional inferiority and chemical infliction that I now feel we need to 'boost' our juice if we cannot get home/locally-grown organic produce.

Superfoods

There is another reason to 'boost your juice'. This is when we are looking at fruits, plants and herbs that we cannot juice or get hold of. The best examples are the amazing superfoods goji berries and acai, which have been heralded as the finest sources of antioxidants on the planet. These are grown thousands of miles away and perish far too quickly to be transported to us in their fresh state. For this reason we can buy these superfoods after they have been dried at low temperatures to preserve pretty much most of their enzyme activity and life force.

Another superfood is spirulina, arguably one of the healthiest foods on the planet. A form of algae comprising 60 per cent protein, it is bursting with essential vitamins, minerals, phytonutrients, antioxidants, betacarotene and essential fatty acids. It provides an amazing boost to your body's natural defence system as, amongst other things, it is reported to be the world's best source of betacarotene, containing 10 times more than its nearest rival, the carrot.

Boosters and Supplements

A booster can be used to lean on during times when you simply cannot juice. On these occasions you can simply mix the powders with water or shop-bought cloudy organic apple juice to top up your health bank account. There is a multitude of herbs, grasses, berries and algae that are beneficial for the above reasons. This is why I have developed a small range of juice boosters and supplements containing all the vegetation I feel the body can benefit from. These 100 per cent natural, vegan powders have been designed to be taken alongside juicing to make up for the shortfall in nutrient content of much of today's produce.

Health is not an area for compromise.

One of the main reasons for developing my own range was, once again, to get rid of some of the rubbish out there. They are often more expensive than most, but health is not an area for compromise. Again, you get what you pay for. Because the boosters can be pricy, I have produced an economical 'variety pack' so people can test them without it costing the earth. After my last book, I was criticized by some people for suggesting that readers use supplements to boost their seven-day juice and smoothie diet. Some people thought I was making this suggestion because I sold the supplements on my website. They chose to ignore the fact that I sold a range which wasn't my own, and that I mentioned other suppliers too.

During the launch programme, the only extra 'boost' you will require is spirulina. However, any of the juices and smoothies can be 'boosted'. Unless you're using organic, locally/home-grown produce I would recommended boosting at least one of your juices or smoothies per day. I always boost my juice to ensure my health investment is strong.

You can, however, *Juice Yourself Slim* without using the boosters. What is more, please feel free to source your own boosters and supplements, although make sure you are not paying for expensive fillers and that they are pulverized to a fine powder so that they mix thoroughly with water or juice. Much more information can be found on juicemaster.com

JUICE YOURSELF SLIM RECIPES

The average person will make just two recipes from a recipe book. It appears that Jamie and Gordon may well be part of the modern kitchen, but the chances of any of their often delicious recipes actually appearing on a plate seem slim. If we all ate more at home from fresh ripe ingredients, as the boys suggest, perhaps we wouldn't be in the health and fat situation we are in.

Luckily, this isn't a recipe book. It's not colourful or glossy, and there aren't any nice pictures in it. This is an information, psychology and self-health book (if you will). As such, you will have many more reasons to make the following recipes than simply trying to impress at a dinner party! I have also added nutritional highlights about every recipe to give you even more incentive to make them.

All of the recipes needed for the launch can be found here plus a large selection of juicy extras. You would no doubt expect all the juice and smoothie recipes to be gorgeous and nutritionally balanced, but you may be surprised at just how delicious and healthy the salads and soups are too.

14

Super-slimming Juices

Here you will find some amazing recipes using some of the finest ingredients from Mother Nature's generously stocked larder. These freshly extracted fruit and vegetable juices provide some of the best refreshment and nutrition on the planet. This chapter is full of cleverly combined recipes with just the right hint of ginger or twist of lime. All the juices contain 100-per-cent natural ingredients with no artificial anything.

Freshly extracted juices provide the body with an array of vitamins, minerals, antioxidants, enzymes and amino acids. These amazing properties, plus the intangible 'X-factor', have an unquantifiable effect on your health. All the scientific research in the world cannot fully explain nature's amazing ability to protect, heal and nourish when food is taken in its natural state.

As well as naturally providing the body with everything it needs on a cellular level to really help *Juice Yourself Slim*, these juices do a whole lot more for your system. Unlike all prescription and non-prescription drugs, which can inflict a multitude of negative side-effects on the body, juicing initiates the complete opposite. During the seven-day launch programme you will experience subtle changes in your body from increased energy levels to weight loss, glowing skin and bright eyes. As you continue juicing yourself slim *for life* you will probably notice more significant changes such as reduced blood pressure levels as well as improvements with conditions such as osteoporosis and arthritis.

The power of juicing is not to be underestimated. While you may have bought this book simply to shed a few pounds, by the time you embark on your new juicy journey *for life* you too will be singing juicing's many virtues from the roof tops. So get your juicer out and start generating some of the best natural medicine on the planet.

Beta-Carrot Juice

'Rich vibrant beetroot combined with sweet carrots and parsnip creates a truly scrummy, nutrient-packed juice.'

2 **apples**
½ **beetroot**
2 small **carrots**
1 small **parsnip**
¼ **lemon** (unwaxed if possible, with the skin on)
ice

1. Juice the apples, beetroot, carrots, parsnip and lemon (pack the lemon between the other produce).
2. Pour over ice and enjoy.

How will it juice me to health? The use of carrots in the fight against cancer has been well-documented due to their high betacarotene content and the presence of the natural fungicide falcarinol. Beetroot is a great source of iron, which means it helps purify the blood. This juice is superb for helping to build the blood and is great for fighting infections. Despite some of the 'earthy' ingredients, the apple, beetroot and carrots actually have a sweet flavour, which work together to create a delicious juice.

Green Slimming Fuel

'Nature's dark, rich, green leafy vegetables, combined with sweet pineapple, create a gorgeous juice packed with Mother Nature's finest goodness.'

⅓ medium **pineapple** (with the skin on)
1 cm **broccoli** stem
Large handful of **spinach**
Handful of **watercress**
Handful of **kale**
¼ **courgette**
¼ **cucumber**
¼ **lime** (with the skin on)
ice

1. Juice all the ingredients, packing the spinach, watercress, kale and lime between the other produce.
2. Pour over ice and enjoy.

How will it juice me to health? If in doubt on the health front, 'green' is where it's at. Green chlorophyll-rich plants use the energy from the sun and convert it into food energy. These vegetables contain an array of amino acids, enzymes, vitamins, minerals and trace elements. This juice is superb for helping to strengthen the body and fight infections.

To add an extra boost of green fuel ... The best forms of rich chlorophyll super fuel are probably our friends wheatgrass and spirulina, so add a shot to really boost your juice. **Wheatgrass** is best fresh. You can either grow it yourself or buy it in trays. However, you will need a special juicer to extract the juice, so if you don't have the time or inclination then use a *good-quality* wheatgrass powder instead. **Spirulina** is an alga that we cannot juice, so again invest in a *good-quality* supplement (be aware that not all supplements are the same and many are bulked out with inexpensive fillers). Both wheatgrass and spirulina can be found in any good health-food shop or at juicemaster.com

Soup-a-Juice

'So named because the pulp left over from making this juice can be cleverly transformed into a gorgeous soup (page 244) — how soup-er is that!'

2 medium **carrots**
1 **parsnip**
1 **apple**
½ **courgette**
ice

1. Juice the carrots, parsnip, apple and courgette.
2. Pour over ice and enjoy.

Sweet juicy tip This juice has a good earthy taste, which may or may not make it your favourite juice on the planet! If you want to make it sweeter: when you have emptied the pulp into the pan to make the soup, simply juice a couple more apples and add to the juice.

How will it juice me to health? Despite its pale colour, the parsnip is in fact richer in vitamins and minerals than the carrot and has a particularly high concentration of potassium. This juice is great for helping nerve function and maintaining the delicate sodium-potassium balance, which governs the fluid and electrolyte balance in the body.

Soup-a-Juice? To make a delicious soup from the leftover pulp simply follow the juicy instructions on page 244. It's important to make up the stock for the soup straight away, before the ingredients oxidize. Once this has cooled it should be placed in the fridge until you are ready to make the soup (use within two days). If you don't make the soup then you can always use the pulp as a great face pack!

Apple 'n' Pear Zesty Twist

'Sweet pear and apple, sharply contrasted with zesty lemon, is nothing short of sublime.'

2 **pears**
2 **apples**
¼ **lemon**, peeled (peel as close to the skin as possible as this is where the majority of this zesty fruit's nutrients are to be found)
ice

1. Juice the pears, apples and lemon, packing the lemon between the other produce.
2. Pour over ice.

How will it juice me to health? Apples are tremendously good for you. Hundreds of studies indicate they can help with numerous aspects of your health. They are renowned for their ability to help flush toxins from the body due to the soluble fibre (pectin) found within the apple. One study has even shown that children who drank apple juice at least once a day were half as likely to suffer from wheezing.

Sweet 'n' Savoury

'Sweet apple and pineapple juice contrasted with earthy spinach and watercress and zinged with a hint of lime.'

2 **apples**
¼ **pineapple**
Handful of **watercress**
Handful of **spinach**
¼ **lime** (with skin on)
ice

1. Juice the apples, pineapple, watercress, spinach and lime by packing the watercress, spinach and lime between the apples.
2. Pour over ice and enjoy.

How will it juice me to health? Watercress and spinach are powerful sources of a range of vitamins and minerals. Watercress is brimming with betacarotene and vitamin A equivalents, which as well as being important antioxidants are also needed for healthy skin and eyes. It is also a fantastic source of vitamins C, B1, B6, K and E, iron, calcium, magnesium, manganese and zinc. Spinach is well-documented for its high concentration of iron and folate. It is particularly helpful if you are pregnant or anaemic. This juice provides a good source of calcium and other alkaline elements essential for retaining blood alkalinity.

Slimlime Tonic

'Pure natural "Slimlime Tonic" without any artificial sweeteners or preservatives — simple yet delicious.'

2 **apples**

1 **lime** (skin removed, but remember to leave on as much of the pith as possible as this is where most of the good stuff is to be found)

1 small bottle (50cl) of lightly sparkling **mineral water** (such as Perrier)

ice

1. Juice the apples and lime into a jug and add the sparkling mineral water.
2. Pour over ice and enjoy this genuine 'Slimlime Tonic'.

How will it juice me slim? This is a superb alternative to the traditional drink and is virtually calorie-free. It also makes an interesting change from mineral water and is a great way to rehydrate the body. It provides the body with vitamins A, B and C as well as a little natural sugar for a quick pick-me-up. Apples are a wonderful fruit, and amongst other things they contain malic acid, which is important to help digest rich, fatty foods. If you are just starting the programme, this will really help to kick-start clearing the system.

Body Balancer

'The natural flavour of sweet pineapple, combined with chlorophyll-rich spinach and the neutral taste of cucumber and celery, makes this a great taste amalgamation as well as a terrific way to neutralize and balance the inner body.'

⅓ medium **pineapple**
1 stick of **celery**
¼ **cucumber**
Handful of **spinach**
ice

1. Juice the pineapple, celery, cucumber and spinach by packing the spinach between the other produce.
2. Pour over ice and enjoy.

How will it balance my body? Celery and cucumber provide the body with a perfect combination of potassium and sodium. Spinach is a good source of calcium and other alkaline elements that are essential to help keep tissues clean and retain blood alkalinity. The combined ingredients in this juice are excellent at helping the body maintain a natural equilibrium.

Why not boost your juice? To make this juice even more balancing and alkaline you could add a teaspoon of the Juice Master's Ultimate Detox Boost, which is packed with ingredients such as milk thistle, parsley, burdock root, red clover and many, many more. This boost really helps to alkalinize the system and enhance the detox process.

Cantaloupe Cooler

'Simple unadulterated pure melon juice is nothing short of divine!'

½ **cantaloupe melon** (washed but not peeled)
ice

1. Cut the melon into sections and juice the entire fruit – yes, even the skin as this is where the real magic is found in terms of nutritional value. The juicer is a clever bit of kit that can happily extract the juice from the flesh and reject the pips and skin.
2. Pour over ice and enjoy.

How will it juice me to health? This juice tastes absolutely divine and is so good for rehydrating the system. Cantaloupes are an excellent source of vitamin A due to their high betacarotene content that gets converted to vitamin A inside the body. This vitamin is renowned for its effect on vision, and studies have shown that people with a diet rich in vitamin A have a reduced risk of developing cataracts. Cantaloupe is also a terrific source of vitamin C, which means this juice is also wonderful for helping to boost the immune system and mop up free radical damage.

Spinach Stout

'This juice genuinely looks like stout, or Guinness, as it has the same thick creamy head. However, the juice is a magnificent deep green colour and contains a whole lot more than just a good supply of iron.'

2 large handfuls of **baby spinach**
¼ **pineapple**
¼ **cucumber**
1 medium **carrot**
⅓ **lemon**, peeled
ice

1. Juice the spinach, pineapple, cucumber, carrot and lemon by packing the spinach and lemon between the other produce.
2. Pour over ice and enjoy.

How will it juice me to health? Many people have traditionally drunk Guinness for its, hmm, 'iron content' believing – or choosing to believe – that 'Guinness is good for you.' Although Guinness does contain about 0.3mg of iron per pint, it really is not the best source due to the alcohol and other chemicals it contains. You will get far, far more iron from consuming fruits and vegetables than you will from downing even 10 pints of Guinness. This version is 100 per cent healthy and genuinely 'good for you', containing an awesome amount of vitamins and minerals as well as, of course, a readily bio-available supply of iron!

Cucumber, Apple 'n' Kiwi Cooler

'The fresh mellow taste of cucumber, apple and kiwi makes this a truly refreshing sensation.'

½ **cucumber** (with the skin on)
1 **kiwi** (remove the skin)
2 **apples**
ice

1. Juice the cucumber, kiwi and apples.
2. Pour over ice and enjoy.

How will it juice me to health? Apples are great for helping to remove impurities in the body, as the pectin found within them acts as an 'intestinal broom'. Cucumbers are fantastic for cooling the inner body and rehydrating the system.

Kiwis are packed with vitamin C. In fact, they contain far more pound for pound than oranges. Vitamin C is excellent for neutralizing free radicals that can cause damage to cells and lead to problems such as inflammation and cancer. A good intake of vitamin C has been shown to be helpful in reducing the severity of conditions like osteoarthritis, rheumatoid arthritis and asthma, and for preventing conditions such as colon cancer, atherosclerosis and diabetic heart disease.

This juice is great for the liver and kidneys as well as for the hair, nails and skin and immune system.

Juicy note Kiwis can be juiced with the skin on. However, this can sometimes leave a harsh taste in the back of the throat, depending on the tartness of the kiwi.

Carrot 'n' Pineapple Twist

'The simple combination of freshly extracted pineapple, carrot and lemon juice creates a delicious, vibrant taste.'

2 **carrots**
¼ **pineapple**
¼ **lemon** (unwaxed with the skin on)
ice

1. Juice the carrots, pineapple and lemon by packing the lemon between the other produce.
2. Pour over ice and enjoy.

How will it juice me to health? Carrots are famous for both their betacarotene content and their ability to help with night vision. The high betacarotene content of the humble carrot has been heralded for centuries as one of the best forms of cancer prevention, and carrot juice is recommended to help the liver cleanse itself. Carrots also contain a good array of nutrients from potassium and magnesium through to vitamins B, C, E and K. Pineapple also contains potassium, an important mineral for healthy muscle and nerve function. The pineapple is a unique source of bromelain, a powerful enzyme that encourages the secretion of hydrochloric acid to help digest protein.

Pear, Pineapple and Ginger Juice

'Thick, naturally sweet pear and creamy pineapple juice contrast with the sharp taste of fresh ginger.'

2 firm **pears**
¼ large **pineapple**
1 cm cube of **ginger**
ice

1. Juice the pears, pineapple and ginger by packing the ginger between the other produce.
2. Pour over ice and enjoy.

How will it juice me slim? Pear juice is lovely and thick and naturally sweet, so this juice will fill you up whilst satisfying your sweet taste buds. Pears also contain pectin, a soluble fibre that can help the body flush out toxins. This juice provides a good source of vitamin C and copper, which both help protect cells from free-radical damage. Vitamin C is critical for good immune function and stimulates white cells to fight infection, directly killing many bacteria and viruses. What's more, pineapple contains bromelain, an enzyme that aids digestion, so this juice will be very easily digested, allowing the body more energy for other activities such as weight loss.

Sweet Veggie Heaven

'Zesty lemon and sharp ginger combined with the natural sweetness of pineapple and apple juice and balanced by the cool savoury tastes of fresh water-rich vegetables.'

3 **apples**
1 stick of **celery**
¼ **courgette**
¼ **cucumber**
¼ **yellow pepper**
¼ **lemon**, peeled
1 cm **ginger** (with the skin on)
ice

1. Juice the apples, celery, courgette, cucumber, pepper, lemon and ginger by packing the lemon and ginger between the other produce.
2. Pour over ice and enjoy.

How will it juice me to health? This juice contains a diverse combination of nutrients including vitamins A, B, C and E and minerals calcium, chlorine, copper, iron, magnesium, phosphorus, potassium, sulphur, sodium and silica.

The cucumber and celery are natural diuretics, so are great for reducing fluid retention. They also contain sodium and potassium, which is crucial for the movement of fluid between cells and fundamental to many bodily processes. These vegetables are also very good for helping to maintain the body's delicate pH balance, which can often become too acidic due to a poor diet.

The apple and lemon are both very cleansing to the system. The acid found within the lemon helps to eliminate toxins in the intestinal tract, and the soluble fibre (pectin) in the apple forms a type of gel that literally 'sweeps' toxins out of the intestines.

Orchard Delight

'Sweet crisp apple and naturally thick pear juice combined with the delightful flavour of freshly squeezed grapes.'

2 **apples**
1 handful of **grapes** (red or white)
2 **pears**
ice

1. Juice the apples, grapes and pears by packing the grapes between the other produce.
2. Pour over ice and enjoy.

How will it juice me to health? Grapes have a high mineral content that helps restore the alkaline balance of the system. They are also great for good bowel movement and proper kidney function. Most importantly, grapes have a high antioxidant content and contain polyphenols, which are the main reason why it is said 'red wine is good for the heart'. Antioxidants are really important for mopping up free radicals, which can create all sorts of damage in the body from premature aging of the skin through to heart disease and cancer. Freshly extracted grape juice is far superior to the fermented bottled version and a much better source of antioxidants and live enzyme activity. So if you're drinking wine simply to get your antioxidants then you might as well start eating Jaffa Cakes to get your vitamin C!

Pepper Punch

'The distinctive taste of freshly juiced peppers and beetroot, sweetened naturally by delicious apples and the added punch of zesty lemon.'

2 **apples**
½ **red pepper**, deseeded
½ **yellow pepper**, deseeded
1 small raw **beetroot**
½ **lemon**, peeled
ice

1. Juice the apples, peppers, beetroot and lemon by packing the lemon between the other produce.
2. Pour over ice and enjoy.

How will it juice me to health? Beetroot is exceptional for helping to rebuild red blood cells and prevent iron deficiencies (anaemia). The high levels of betacarotene in this juice help to mop up free radical damage which can otherwise cause a multitude of diseases in the body. Peppers are high in vitamins B and C and are also a source of capsaicin, a natural painkiller thought to be beneficial for arthritic pain.

This juice contains fruit and vegetables from across the colour spectrum. In fact, the different phytochemicals and antioxidants in the fruits and vegetables give them their colour. According to the *British Medical Journal*, if you consume a range of produce from across the colour spectrum every day, 'you will receive the perfect cocktail of phytochemicals, vitamins and minerals'.

Fruity Rescue Remedy

'This array of citrus fruits and tropical pineapple provides a totally refreshing juice that will quench your thirst, zing your taste buds and boost your immune system.'

2 **oranges**, peeled*
¼ **lemon**, peeled*
½ **lime**, peeled*
⅓ medium **pineapple**
ice

* With the citrus fruits, make sure that when you peel them you leave as much of the pith on as possible as this is where the majority of the vitamins are to be found.

1. Juice the oranges, lemon, lime and pineapple by packing the lemon and lime between the other produce.
2. Pour over ice and enjoy.

How will it juice me to health? This juice contains a good supply of vitamin C found in the oranges, lemon and lime. Vitamin C is an important antioxidant involved in the development of connective tissues, lipid metabolism, immune function and wound healing. An extreme lack of vitamin C can lead to the disease scurvy. Thousands of mariners used to die from scurvy until the humble lemon came to the rescue. Today, vitamin C is more renowned for its ability to help boost the immune system and is often used to fight off the common cold. So whenever you're feeling a little under the weather make yourself a glass of Fruity Rescue Remedy.

A Very Tarty Tonic

'The tartness of freshly juiced cranberries is cleverly mellowed by the natural sweetness of apple, pineapple and pear juice.'

1 handful of **cranberries**
1 **apple**
1 **pear**
½ medium **pineapple**
ice

1. Juice the cranberries, apple, pear and pineapple by packing the cranberries between the other produce.
2. Pour over ice and enjoy.

How will it juice me to health? Cranberries are renowned for their ability to help clear up bladder infections. This is because they contain an antibacterial agent that prevents *E. coli* from sticking to the walls of the urinary tract. What is more, they contain a strong acid called quinine which helps to remove toxins from the bladder, kidneys, prostate and testicles. Pears and apples are both good for flushing out toxins as they contain pectin, a soluble fibre that effectively forms a gel in the intestines which carries away toxins.

Pineapple 'n' Cinnamon Spice

'Freshly extracted, creamy and delicious pineapple juice blended with mellow sweet apple juice and complemented by spicy, warming cinnamon.'

2 **apples**
¼ medium **pineapple**
1 small teaspoon of **cinnamon**
ice

1. Juice the apples and pineapple.
2. Pour into a blender along with the cinnamon and ice.

Juicy tip If you don't have a blender you can simply stir the cinnamon into the juice, although you need to do it quite vigorously to avoid any little lumps.

How will it juice me to health? Pineapples contain a powerful enzyme called bromelain which encourages the secretion of hydrochloric acid. This is a very useful enzyme for digesting protein, which is why meats such as gammon are often served alongside pineapple. Cinnamon is a clever little spice. It contains the compound cinnamaldehyde which prevents unwanted clumping of blood platelets that could otherwise cause blood clotting. Cinnamon could also significantly help people with type 2 diabetes to normalize their blood sugar levels. Studies have shown that compounds found in cinnamon not only stimulate insulin receptors, but also inhibit an enzyme that inactivates them, thus significantly increasing the cell's ability to use glucose and regulate blood sugar levels.

Purple Power

'Vibrant, rich, decadent grapes and blueberries, freshly squeezed with pure natural apple juice, create a purple elixir that tastes just blissful.'

1 large handful of **red grapes**
1 large handful of **blueberries**
2 **apples**
ice

1. Juice the grapes, blueberries and apples by packing the grapes and blueberries between the apples.
2. Pour over ice and enjoy.

What's the juicy science? Blueberries are one of the richest sources of antioxidants available to us. In fact, they are one of the most nutrient-dense foods on the planet. Two of the phytochemicals found in blueberries – anthocyanins and phenolics – are constantly being studied for their anti-aging and anti-cancer benefits. This magical supply of antioxidants has many other profound health benefits for the body, from helping to maintain cholesterol levels to supporting a healthy urinary tract.

Grapes also contain a selection of wondrous nutrients known as polyphenols, some of the most potent plant antioxidants in nature. These compounds protect the plants from disease; studies are suggesting they can do the same for the human body. The *Anti-Cancer Research Journal* indicated that the polyphenol resveratrol 'appears to exhibit anti-cancer properties by its ability to suppress proliferation of a wide variety of tumour cells'.

This juice is therefore excellent for furnishing your body with disease-fighting super troops!

The World's Your Oyster

'The cool neutral flavours of celery, cucumber and mangetout are deepened by the earthy tastes of spinach, watercress and broccoli and sweetened by creamy, decadent fresh pineapple and sweet apple.'

1 small handful of **spinach**
1 small handful of **watercress**
1 cm of **broccoli** stem
1 stick of **celery**
¼ **cucumber**
1 small handful of **mangetout**
¼ medium **pineapple**
2 **apples**
ice

1. Juice the spinach, watercress, broccoli, celery, cucumber, mangetout, pineapple and apples by packing the spinach, watercress and mangetout between the other produce.
2. Pour over ice and enjoy.

How will it juice me to health? There are so many vitamins, minerals, phytonutrients and antioxidants in this juice it would be simply impossible to name them all. It is sufficient to say that this juice is crammed with goodness including the special 'X factor' – chlorophyll – that is found in all the rich green vegetables. Chlorophyll has a similar molecular structure to haemoglobin, the part of the blood which carries oxygen around the body. In a similar way, chlorophyll helps to oxygenate the bloodstream and this has a multitude of beneficial effects on the body.

A Juicy Special This juice was created by a very special chap called Dan and his father Allen, whom I had the good fortune to meet at The Good Food Show. Happy juicing guys – the world really is your oyster!

15

Super-slimming Smoothies

Thick, creamy smoothies with decadent, divine tastes and delicious aromas that will make your taste buds dance and your tummy sing – that's what these recipes are all about.

Once you have become acquainted with some of these recipes you will realize there is no need for artificial flavours or colours or added sugars and fats to create something that looks and tastes incredible. Nature has provided us with a whole menu of delightful ingredients that, when combined in a specific way, create something every bit as enjoyable as a *Triple Diple Death by Chocolate* dessert (yes, the clue is in the name) but without any of the calorie-crammed fats, insulin-robbing and diabetes-inducing refined sugars or mind-altering artificial colours or flavours.

The main difference between a smoothie and a juice is that a smoothie contains the whole fruit/vegetable blended together with fruit/vegetable juice, whereas a juice is simply the pure liquid extracted from the fruit or vegetable. A smoothie therefore contains the fibre of the fruit and can also have things like yoghurt, seeds, nuts and honey added, so it is much more filling and a genuine meal in a glass. On this note, please drink your smoothies slowly as they can contain a lot of whole foods. Your body is not used to swallowing down a whole banana and a handful of berries all in one gulp. Just enjoy the drink and treat it as you would any other meal.

All these smoothies are made with 100 per cent natural ingredients, and there is a great balance of both vegetable and fruit smoothies. All the vegetable-based smoothies contain avocado, a much misunderstood little fruit (yes, an avocado is a fruit, not a vegetable). Avocados have received some very unfair press, propagated by certain 'diet' clubs, and have been tarnished the 'devil food' of the slimming world. I have only one thing to say to this: **'RUBBISH!'** Avocados contain EFAs (essential fatty acids), which are excellent for the body. These 'good' fats actually help to regulate and suppress the appetite. This can reduce cravings for sugary, fattening foods. What's more, the 'good' fats act as a buffer to prevent the quick release of any fruit sugars into the bloodstream. So, contrary to some misguided beliefs, avocados are **REALLY** important for this weight-loss programme.

All the smoothies found in this chapter are super healthy and super slimming, so get your blender warmed up and prepare to smoothie yourself slim!

Fruity Superfood Sensation

'Plump blueberries and ripe banana combined with the divine flavours of freshly extracted pomegranate and orange juice.'

2 **oranges**
⅙ **lemon** with the skin on (unwaxed if possible)
2 tablespoons of **blueberries**
½ **banana**
1 small handful of **goji berries** (either dried or powdered, see note on page 203)
1 **pomegranate**
ice

1. Juice the oranges and lemon and pour into a blender.
2. Add the blueberries, banana, goji berries, pomegranate juice *(see note on page 203)* and ice.
3. Blend until smooth.

Juicy notes To get the 'good stuff' from pomegranates can be somewhat difficult. I'm sure we all have memories of desperately trying to remove those little 'pips' with a sharp needle? Even the most sophisticated electric juicer cannot get the 'good stuff' from this amazing fruit. Instead, you will need an old-fashioned citrus juicer which will allow you to place half the pomegranate against the juicer and apply enough pressure to extract some juice. If you do not have such a juicer (or the inclination), you can omit pomegranate from this recipe.

How will this make me super? Superfoods are dense in a wide variety of nutrients. However, they tend to have a very high concentration of one particular vitamin or mineral. For example, by weight, goji berries contain roughly 500 times the amount of vitamin C in an orange!

To make this extra super ... There are some amazing berries that you simply cannot get fresh in many countries, such as goji berries and acai found in the Himalayas and Amazon rainforest. Once picked they perish very quickly, so the only way for us to experience these amazing berries is for them to be dried or pulped as soon as they are picked, thus preserving their amazing life force. Just like in the desert, as soon as liquid is applied – boom! These little babies come to life along with all their amazing health properties.

You can buy dried goji berries from any good health-food shop or get hold of a good-quality powdered booster (watch out for expensive fillers). The Juice Master's Berry Boost contains 100 per cent berries including fruits such as goji berries, acai, pomegranate, blueberries and many more superfoods, so add a spoonful to make this smoothie extra 'super'.

Savoury Superfood Sensation

'Delicious, creamy, sweet pineapple blends beautifully with this host of superfood vegetables to create a great tasting and extraordinary smoothie.'

¼ ripe **avocado**
ice
1 small piece of **broccoli** stem
1 handful of **spinach**
1 handful of **sprouts** (not Brussels sprouts, cause they are just WRONG, but sprouted seeds, such as alfalfa and mung beans)
¼ **pineapple**
⅙ **lemon** with the skin on (unwaxed if possible)

1. Place the avocado flesh and ice into a blender.
2. Juice the broccoli, spinach, sprouts, pineapple and lemon and pour into the blender.
3. Blend until smooth.

How will superfoods get me 'juiced'? Superfoods are dense in a wide variety of nutrients. They often contain not just vitamins, minerals and phytonutrients but also a range of essential fatty acids and amino acids. Genuine superfoods are so super that it is alleged you could survive on them solely and get all your nutritional requirements, but hey! We believe variety is important.

Sprouts are one of the few vegetables that gain vitamins after they have been harvested because they continue to grow. So sprouts are super good for you.

To make this extra super ... There are some amazing plants and herbs that you either cannot get a lot of juice from or you simply cannot get hold of. What's more, intensive farming has depleted a lot of the vital vitamins and minerals from the soil, so it is always a good idea to boost your juice or smoothie every now and again. For this reason I have developed a really funky range of boosters and supplements packed with things like spirulina, wheatgrass, barley grass, alfalfa, friendly bacteria and much, much more.

If you really want to make this smoothie extra super, add a shot of The Juice Master's Ultimate Juice Boost.

Organic Avocado Crush

'Creamy ripe organic avocado blended with freshly extracted pineapple juice and a twist of lime.'

½ ripe organic **avocado**
ice – lots of it
½ medium **pineapple**
1 peeled **lime**

1. Place the avocado flesh and ice into a blender.
2. Juice the pineapple and lime by packing the lime in between the pineapple.
3. Pour this juice into the blender and blend until smooth.

How will it juice me to health? Pineapple juice has anti-inflammatory properties and powerful enzymes that aid the digestion of protein. It is said to be good for arthritis. The strong enzymes and acid can help break down mucus so it is really good for asthma sufferers too. Avocados contain all your nutritional needs, including EFAs (essential fatty acids). Studies have shown that monounsaturated fats, like the ones found in avocados, help reduce cholesterol levels and maintain a healthy heart. Did you know *The Guinness Book of Records* claims that avocados are 'the most nutritious of all fruits'? These little beauties are unbelievable and I personally eat/smoothie as many as I can, whenever I am genuinely hungry.

What about an extra juice boost? To boost the nutritional content of this smoothie you could add a teaspoon of The Juice Master's Ultimate Juice Boost or Ultimate Superfood. This is by no means a necessity, especially if you are using good organic produce. However, if your produce is a little old and inferior then a booster of some description is extremely beneficial.

Blueberry Power

'Plump, rich blueberries, fresh bio-live yoghurt and the sweet juice of crisp apples, all blended together with nature's finest manuka honey.'

2 tablespoons of **blueberries**
3 tablespoons of **bio-live yoghurt** (Yeo Valley do a great one, which is genuinely 98 per cent fat-free with no added sugars)
Squeeze of **manuka honey**
ice
2 **apples**

1. Place the blueberries, yoghurt, honey and ice in a blender.
2. Juice the apples then add this juice to the blender.
3. Blend until smooth.

How will this 'power' my body? Blueberries are an excellent source of antioxidants, folic acid, ellagic acid, betacarotene and vitamins B and C. All these are wonderful for preventing free-radical damage and enhancing the skin's radiance. Bio-live yoghurt contains 'live' cultures which help furnish the gut with friendly bacteria to aid digestion. This smoothie is therefore great for the internal system as well as the external appearance. It's so scrummy it even makes an appearance as a 'special guest' in our Juice 'n' Smoothie Bars!

Ginger Orange Smoothie

'Fresh juicy sweet oranges contrasted with the sharp zing of ginger and softened by the creamy mellow flavour of ripe banana.'

1 **banana**
ice
3 **oranges**, peeled (peel as close to the rind as possible as the majority of nutrients are found directly under the skin)
1 small piece of **ginger**, with the skin on

1. Put the banana and ice in a blender.
2. Juice the oranges and ginger by placing the ginger in between the oranges.
3. Pour the juice into the blender and blend until smooth.

How will it juice me to health? Oranges are rich in vitamins A, B and C as well as calcium and folate. Vitamin C plays a vital role in combating infections, keeping gums healthy and healing wounds. Ginger is a natural decongestant and antibiotic, so these two ingredients are excellent if your immune system is under stress.

Cucumber Shake

'Cool cucumber blended with the freshly extracted juice of delicate apples and courgette, complemented with a twist of earthy spinach and zesty lemon.'

¼ **cucumber**, peeled
ice
2 **apples**
1 handful of **spinach**
¼ **courgette**
¼ **lemon**, peeled (keep as much of the pith on as possible, or if you use unwaxed lemons then leave the skin on for extra zest)

1. Place the cucumber and ice into a blender.
2. Juice the apples, spinach, courgette and lemon by packing the spinach and lemon in between the apples.
3. Pour the juice into a blender and blend really thoroughly until smooth.*

* Please note: depending on the quality of your blender this shake may be smooth or it may have a more 'bitty' consistency — but hey! You might be glad of something you can actually chew!

How will it juice me slim? This shake is incredibly filling and contains a good source of dietary fibre because the cucumber is blended instead of juiced. Cucumbers and courgettes have similar properties as they are from the same 'family'. They are high in vitamins A and C, folic acid and potassium. Cucumbers are renowned as diuretics, so they are great for helping the body to cleanse the kidneys. They also contain silica, which is good for the skin and helps prevent fluid retention. Spinach is a 'wonder food' and one of the best vegetable sources of folate, which helps produce new cells in the body and is particularly needed during times of growth and repair. It is well known that folate is important during pregnancy and infancy. However, it is also fundamental for producing red blood cells and preventing anaemia, no matter what age you are.

Blood Builder

'The juice of vibrant raw beetroot, sweet betacarotene-packed carrots and zesty lemon all blended together with the subtle flavours of creamy avocado.'

¼ **avocado**
ice
2 **apples**
½ raw **beetroot**
2 small **carrots**
¼ **lemon**, peeled (keep as much of the pith on as possible or, if you use unwaxed lemons, keep the skin on for extra zest)

1. Place the avocado flesh and ice into a blender.
2. Juice the apples, beetroot, carrots and lemon by packing the lemon in between the apples.
3. Pour the juice into a blender and blend until smooth.

How will it build my body? Beetroot is exceptional at helping to rebuild blood cells and for assisting the body with cleansing the bloodstream. Carrots are betacarotene kings and contain many vital vitamins, minerals and phytonutrients. The high levels of betacarotene in this smoothie help mop up free radicals that could otherwise create havoc in your system. Free radicals are caused by stress, environmental pollution, nicotine, alcohol and even over-exercising (bummer, huh?). The X-factor contained within fruits and vegetables can be viewed as the free-radical police, which work to neutralize free-radical damage. This is one of those really amazing smoothies, which will do more good for your body than we will ever really know.

Strawberry and Mango Melt

'Succulent strawberries combined with mouth-watering mango, delicious freshly extracted apple juice and creamy bio-live yoghurt.'

½ **mango**, peeled and de-stoned
1 handful of **strawberries**
2 tablespoons of **bio-live yoghurt** (Yeo Valley do a really creamy one, which is genuinely 98 per cent fat-free with no added sugars)
ice
2 **apples**

1. Place the mango flesh, strawberries, yoghurt and ice in a blender.
2. Juice the apples and pour this juice into the blender.
3. Blend until smooth.

How will it juice me slim? The gorgeous combination of blended mango, strawberries and yoghurt creates a particularly thick smoothie which will make your tummy feel content and satisfy even the sweetest taste buds. This smoothie is loaded with minerals – zinc, iron, calcium and potassium – and vitamins A, B and C. It has particularly high levels of potassium, which is important for maintaining a healthy nervous system and for controlling the fluid balance in the body. Strawberries are full of vitamin C as well as a host of antioxidants and are really helpful in supporting the immune system. The bio-live yoghurt contains a variety of friendly bacteria that furnish the gut and help digestion as well as fight bacterial infections.

Rocket Fuel

'The unique flavour of wild rocket combined with mild celery, creamy avocado and sweet apples creates an unusual yet delicious smoothie.'

¼ ripe **avocado**
ice
2 **apples**
1 stick of **celery**
¼ **cucumber**
1 handful of **wild rocket**

1. Place the avocado flesh and ice into a blender.
2. Juice the apples, celery, cucumber and rocket by packing the rocket in between the apples.
3. Pour the juice into the blender and blend until smooth.

How will it 'rocket' me to health? Wild rocket is a rich source of iron as well as vitamins A and C, folate and calcium. The phytochemicals that give rocket its bright green colour and distinctive flavour also help the body fight against disease. Avocados are an excellent source of carbohydrate and contain a multitude of nutritious benefits, including essential fatty acids (EFAs). These 'good' fats are, as suggested by the name, essential for the human body. However, the body cannot make them so it is vital that we obtain them through our diet. EFAs are crucial because they support the cardiovascular, reproductive, immune and nervous systems. Unfortunately, many people have a diet very low in EFAs; this can lead to various health problems and has also been linked to depression. So give your body and mind a real launch with this 'Rocket Fuel' smoothie.

Fennel Fuel

'The unique flavour of fresh fennel, sweet pineapple and zesty lime creates a truly refreshing, delicious smoothie.'

¼ ripe **avocado**
ice
⅓ medium **pineapple**
2cm of fresh **fennel**
¼ **cucumber**
½ **lime**, peeled

1. Place the avocado flesh and ice into a blender.
2. Juice the pineapple, fennel, cucumber and lime by packing the fennel and lime in between the pineapple.
3. Pour the juice into the blender and blend until smooth.

How will this 'fuel' my system? Fennel has been used to aid digestive ailments since as far back as the early Egyptians, and many recent studies also support this claim. What's more, fennel has a reputation as an appetite suppressant, so this juice could not only help reduce bloating, stomach cramps and IBS, but also help control the appetite.

Fruity Bio-live Breakfast Smoothie

'Crunchy muesli smothered in creamy bio-live yoghurt and blended with yummy berries and freshly extracted apple juice.'

2 **apples**
1 handful of **muesli**
2 tablespoons of **bio-live yoghurt** (Yeo Valley do a delicious 98 per cent fat-free version with no added sugars)
2 tablespoons of **mixed berries** (fresh or frozen, such as strawberries, blueberries, raspberries)
ice

1. Juice the apples and pour into a blender along with the muesli, yoghurt, mixed berries and ice.
2. Blend as much or as little as you like, depending on required consistency. Personally, I like it fairly crunchy so you can still taste the muesli. However, some people prefer it obliterated to a silky smooth consistency – the choice is all yours!

How will it juice me to health? A good muesli can be packed with an array of whole grains, fruits, seeds, oats and nuts. It can offer a range of vitamins and minerals, complex carbohydrates, fibre, omega 3, 6 and 9, antioxidants and phytoestrogens. Bio-live yoghurt is wonderful for furnishing the body with friendly bacteria that help aid digestion and maintain a healthy gut. The vibrant colour of berries means they contain a host of phytochemicals, which help the body fight against disease by combating free-radical damage. They are also wonderful for helping to promote healthy, glowing skin.

This smoothie is genuinely filling as it really is a meal in a glass – a superb way to start the morning.

Super Sporty Fuel Smoothie

'Freshly extracted sweet apple juice and neutral cucumber blended with creamy ripe banana and avocado.'

½ **banana**
¼ **avocado**
ice
2 **apples**
½ **cucumber**

1. Place the banana, avocado flesh and ice into a blender.
2. Juice the apples and cucumber and add this juice to the blender.
3. Blend until smooth.
4. Drink immediately. This smoothie isn't suitable for making up in advance.

How will it super fuel me? The banana and avocado provide a supreme supply of potassium, which is vital for the nervous system, correct muscle function and fluid balance. This is of particular relevance to any athlete about to undergo an endurance activity. This isn't just rhetoric – go to the start of any marathon and you will find more bananas than are stocked in your local supermarket. The reason bananas are there instead of avocados is simply because they are easier to eat. In fact, avocados contain far more potassium than bananas, and are an awesome source of essential fatty acids (EFAs). 'Good' fats or EFAs are essential for the body, and despite some of the unfair propaganda put out by certain 'diet clubs', they are extremely good for you, **ESPECiALLY** when you are creating a slim, toned, healthy body. The EFAs found in avocados actually help to regulate and suppress the appetite, reducing the craving for sugary, fattening foods. The avocado and banana also act as a buffer so that any natural sugars in this smoothie are released slowly; so this truly provides a slow-releasing source of super fuel for the body and is a must for any athlete.

Cranberry Banana Blend

'Crisp tart cranberries complemented by soft creamy ripe banana and blended with natural sweet pineapple juice.'

½ **banana**
ice
¼ medium **pineapple**
1 **apple**
2 handfuls of fresh or frozen **cranberries**

1. Place the banana and ice into a blender.
2. Juice the pineapple, apple and cranberries by packing the cranberries in between the pineapple.
3. Pour this juice into the blender and blend until smooth.

How will it juice me to health? These little red berries really are one of Mother Nature's remarkable health workers. They are renowned for their ability to help clear up bladder infections because they contain an antibacterial agent that reduces the ability of *E. coli* bacteria to stick to the walls of the urinary tract. Cranberries also contain quinine, an acid that helps remove toxins from the bladder and kidneys as well as the prostate and testicles.

Bio-live Berries

'Decadent sweet juicy berries combined with thick creamy bio-live yoghurt and the juice of freshly extracted pineapple.'

1 large handful of **berries** (use frozen or whatever fresh ones are in season, such as strawberries, blueberries, pitted cherries — expensive but divine! — blackberries)
2 tablespoons of **bio-live yoghurt** (Yeo Valley do a great one, which is genuinely 98 per cent fat-free with no added sugars)
ice
¼ medium **pineapple**

1. Place the berries, yoghurt and ice into a blender.
2. Juice the pineapple, add this juice to the blender and blend until smooth.

How will it juice me to health? Berries are rich in vitamins B, C and E and minerals calcium, potassium, iron, magnesium and phosphorus. They are SO, SO good for you and taste absolutely delicious. They have many properties which can be helpful in reducing the signs of aging, such as helping the skin to keep its elasticity and prevent wrinkles. They are also good for maintaining a healthy male reproductive system and generally boosting the immune system.

What about an extra juice boost? To really boost the health properties of this smoothie you could add a teaspoon of The Juice Master's Ultimate Berry Boost. This contains blueberries, acai, goji berries, pomegranate, cherry juice and other wonderful berries that offer a multitude of health benefits that, due to their ellagic acid and antioxidant content, are particularly good for the skin.

Spirulina Smoothie

'The mighty mineral-packed spirulina, blended with the juice from nature's finest green fruits and vegetables and combined with the flesh of ripe, creamy avocado.'

½ **avocado** (organic if possible)
1 small teaspoon of **spirulina***
ice
2 **apples**
¼ **cucumber**
½ stick of **celery**
1 handful of **spinach**

* Spirulina can be bought in any good health-food shop or at juicemaster.com

1. Place the avocado flesh, spirulina and ice into a blender.
2. Juice the apples, cucumber, celery and spinach by packing the spinach in between the apples.
3. Pour this juice into the blender and blend until smooth.

How will it juice me to health? Spirulina is a real superfood containing a mighty collaboration of goodness. It is packed with essential amino acids – the building bricks for protein – and is also reported to contain 10 times more calcium than milk and 58 times more iron than spinach. What's more, it is bursting with vitamins, minerals, phytonutrients and EFAs (essential fatty acids), and is the betacarotene king, containing around 10 times more than a carrot! It really is a 'wonder food' and, personally, I love its distinctive flavour, but don't be tempted to add too much as it is so potent it could overpower this gorgeous smoothie.

Avocados have such a smooth buttery texture they sometimes taste too good to be healthy! However, they really are terrific for your heart, due to the monounsaturated fats; for your skin, due to the good levels of vitamin E; and for your nerve and muscle function, due to the excellent source of potassium. Avocado is also a great provider of dietary fibre so can help to promote an efficient digestive system.

Mango and Honey Zest

'Fresh ripe banana and mouthwatering mango blended with delicate apple juice, sweet natural honey and zesty lemons.'

½ **banana**
½ **mango**, peeled and de-stoned
Squeeze of **honey**
ice
2 **apples**
⅙ **lemon** with the skin on (if you use an unwaxed lemon leave the skin on for extra zing)

1. Place the banana, mango, honey and ice into a blender.
2. Juice the apples and lemon by packing the lemon in between the apples.
3. Pour the juice into the blender and blend until smooth.

How will it juice me to health? Mangoes supply the body with an array of goodness, including over 20 vitamins and minerals, a multitude of antioxidants, several important enzymes and an ample supply of potassium. Potassium is really important to aid a healthy nervous system and is crucial – alongside the mineral sodium – in regulating the body's water balance. Apples and lemons also contain many vitamins and minerals, including vitamin A – a well-known anti-cancer agent – as well as vitamin C, which is renowned for its ability to promote a healthy immune system.

Natural Skin Boost

'Fresh ripe creamy avocado blended with the juice of cool cucumber, zesty lime and exotic pineapple.'

½ **avocado**
ice
¼ **cucumber**
¼ medium **pineapple**
½ **lime**, peeled

1. Place the avocado flesh and ice into a blender.
2. Juice the cucumber, pineapple and lime by packing the lime in between the pineapple.
3. Pour this juice into the blender and blend until smooth.

How will it boost my skin? Cucumbers are very cooling to the system and help to rehydrate the body and, in turn, the skin. They can also promote elasticity in the skin and have a renowned diuretic effect which helps the body flush toxins from the system. The avocado contains essential fatty acids (EFAs) that are, amongst other things, of paramount importance in creating and maintaining healthy, glowing skin. They are also a great source of zinc, which happens to be one of the best minerals for the skin.

How can i get an extra skin boost? There are a number of key dietary ingredients that can help achieve supreme, healthy, vibrant skin. These include EFAs, zinc, lecithin, selenium, probiotics and red clover. Because you can't often get hold of all these ingredients we have carefully developed our own Clear Skin Booster which contains all the above and more. So if you really need an extra boost, add a teaspoon to your juice or smoothie.

Goji Berry Bonanza

'Wonderful, exotic goji berries, blended with fresh ripe banana, bio-live yoghurt and the juice of sweet crisp apples.'

½ **banana**
1 handful of dried **goji berries***
2 tablespoons of **bio-live yoghurt** (Yeo Valley do a great one, which is genuinely 98 per cent fat-free with no added sugars)
ice
2 **apples**

* You can buy dried goji berries in all good health-food shops, and even Tesco have started stocking them now. However, if you can't get the dried variety you could add a teaspoon of powdered goji berries or The Juice Master's Berry Boost.

1. Place the banana, goji berries, yoghurt and ice into a blender.
2. Juice the apples and pour this juice into the blender.
3. Blend for quite a while until smooth.

How will it juice me to health? Goji berries are the new kids on the block when it comes to hip, must-have foods. A packet of dried goji berries in your shopping basket carries the equivalent status to walking around London with a couple of Abercrombie & Fitch carrier bags. They are right up there with the other highly fashionable 'adjective foods', you know the ones ... 'organic Fair Trade coffee', 'free-range organic mayonnaise', 'omega-3 enriched cereal' and the list goes on. Unlike some of these other foods, goji berries are possibly worth the hype and they will certainly do a lot more for you than any Abercrombie hoodie! They are brimming with goodness and contain more vitamin C than oranges, more iron than a steak and more betacarotene than a carrot. Betacarotene is thought to help fight heart disease, defend against cancer and protect skin from sun damage. I could write an entire book on the health properties of goji berries – and indeed I'm sure someone has – but my philosophy is you don't need to know why they are good for you or exactly what they do for your body; you just need to eat, juice or smoothie them.

Seedy Summer Berry Crush

'Sweet summer strawberries, plump blueberries and nutty sunflower and sesame seeds all blended together with the delicate tones of freshly extracted apple juice.'

1 handful of **strawberries**
1 handful of **blueberries**
1 small handful of **sunflower** and **sesame seeds**
ice
3 **apples**

1. Place the strawberries, blueberries, seeds and ice into a blender.
2. Juice the apples and pour this juice into the blender.
3. Blend.

How will it juice me to health? Sesame and sunflower seeds are great sources of protein, calcium, iron, zinc, magnesium, phosphorus, vitamins B and E as well as EFAs (essential fatty acids). Importantly, sesame and sunflower seeds are rich in cholesterol-lowering phytosterols. These work by inhibiting the incorporation of cholesterol from the gastrointestinal tract, thereby decreasing the amount of cholesterol that is absorbed.

This natural process is so successful that many margarines and butters are now sold as being 'enriched' with phytosterols. You might wonder why we need to take these phytosterols from their natural origin and add them to another food product. Why are we not simply advised to consume more seeds? Oh yes, because the pharmaceutical companies can't make money from us eating more seeds. Pharmaceutical companies pay scientists obscene amounts of money to try and isolate specific health properties from nature so they can make synthetic versions and then sell them to us in a pill or 'enrich' certain foods as a marketing ploy. Nature has so generously given us amazing health properties in all fruits, vegetables, seeds and nuts, and all we need to do is consume them.

Pineapple, Mint and Lime Shake

'Fresh chunks of juicy pineapple blended together with zesty lime, fresh garden mint and the juice of crisp delicate apples.'

¼ medium **pineapple**, peeled and chopped
1 small handful of fresh **mint**
ice
2 **apples**
¼ **lime**, peeled

1. Place the pineapple, mint and ice in a blender.
2. Juice the apples and lime by packing the lime between the apples.
3. Pour this juice into the blender and blend until smooth.

How will it juice me to health? Apples appear so simple yet they are amazing. They contain vitamins A, B and C as well as calcium, chlorine, magnesium, phosphorus, potassium, sulphur and iron. Pectin, a soluble fibre found in apples, works to remove toxins from the intestines. It does this by forming a gel-like substance that quite literally absorbs toxins and flushes them out of the system. Mint is famously good for aiding good digestion and freshening breath. Lime is also a great cleanser, and the strong fruit acids help to eliminate toxins and neutralize harmful bacteria.

Juicy note This smoothie will always have a stringy texture because of the pineapple content. Some people love this, while others are not so keen. If it's too stringy for you, next time simply juice the pineapple as well.

16

Souper Slimming Fuel

Soup can be a much underrated fuel. There is often a big mystery surrounding how to make them as several methods are overcomplicated and can take a long time. In this chapter you will find some amazing soups that can all be made within minutes and contain no butter, milk or cream yet taste absolutely divine.

'Soup-a-juice' is a revolutionary recipe that uses the leftover pulp from the juice to form the basis of the stock for the soup. This is such a neat idea as it means there is zero waste and you are extracting every bit of goodness from your produce. You can have some fun here and play around with other versions, although you might want to use the pulp from the predominantly vegetable juices or you could end up with some very unusual sweet-tasting soups … but who knows – pear, pineapple, ginger and sweet potato soup might just become the next big thing!

THESE RECIPES HAPPILY MAKE ENOUGH FOR TWO PEOPLE, SO WATCH OUT!

Please take note of the above, especially when on the seven day launch. If making for one, either halve the ingredients or store half for the following day. You can genuinely fill up on these soups without any guilt as they are so ridiculously good for you. Each one contains nothing more than a multitude of fresh vegetables, a stock cube and a tablespoon of vegetable oil. All this natural goodness helps to create an excellent health insurance portfolio.

Butternut Squash and Carrot Soup

'Creamy smooth butternut squash and carrot infused together to create a genuinely dreamy, sublime, nourishing soup.'

½ **butternut squash**
3 medium **carrots**
1 small **red onion**
1 **vegetable stock cube**
1 tablespoon of **vegetable oil**
Crushed **black pepper**

1. Peel the butternut squash (remove seeds), carrots and red onion and chop all the vegetables into small chunks.
2. Prepare the stock by dissolving the stock cube in 1 pint (570ml) of boiling water.
3. In a large saucepan heat the oil, add all the vegetables and season with black pepper.
4. Gently sweat the vegetables over a medium heat with the lid on for 15 minutes, stirring occasionally.
5. Add the stock, bring to the boil and simmer for 10 minutes.
6. Remove from the heat and, using a blender (hand or jug), blend the soup until smooth.
7. Pour into a bowl and enjoy.

Why is this soup-a good for me? Carrots are an excellent source of antioxidant compounds, and the richest vegetable source of the pro-vitamin A carotenes. Butternut squash is also an excellent source of vitamin A (in the form of betacarotene) and a very good source of vitamins C, B1, B6 and B3 (niacin), potassium, dietary fibre, manganese, copper, folate and omega-3 fatty acids.

One of the most abundant nutrients in both vegetables, betacarotene has been shown to have powerful antioxidant and anti-inflammatory properties. It is able to protect against cardiovascular disease and strokes as well as help protect the body against cancer. It also promotes good vision, especially night vision.

'Souper' Green Stuff

'The fresh vibrant pure tones of Mother Nature's finest chlorophyll-rich vegetables, all blended together to create a little taste of Eden.'

1 **leek**
1 stick of **celery**
1 **courgette**
1 **vegetable stock cube**
1 tablespoon of **vegetable oil**
6 **broccoli florets**, chopped into small pieces
50g **spinach**
Crushed **black pepper**

1. 'Top and tail' the leek, celery and courgette and chop into thin slices.
2. Prepare the stock by dissolving the stock cube in 1 pint (570ml) of boiling water.
3. In a large saucepan heat the oil, add all the vegetables and season with black pepper.
4. Gently sweat the vegetables over a medium heat for 15 minutes then add the stock and seasoning, bring to the boil and simmer for 5 minutes.
5. Remove from the heat and, using a blender (hand or jug), blend the soup slightly so it retains a good chunky texture.
6. Pour into a bowl and enjoy.

Why is this soup-a good for me? Broccoli is packed with nutrients, including the phytonutrients sulforaphane and the indoles, which have been shown to provide significant anti-cancer properties. Many studies support the beneficial health effects of broccoli, which also include helping to boost the immune system.

Leeks are part of the allium family. A high intake of these vegetables has been shown to reduce total cholesterol and LDL, or 'bad', cholesterol levels while at the same time raising HDL, or 'good', cholesterol levels.

Spinach contains high levels of vitamins A, B, C and K, manganese, folate, iron and calcium. Studies have found that spinach is useful for helping the body fight against osteoporosis, heart disease, colon cancer, arthritis and other diseases.

Tomato and Basil Soup

'The complementary flavours of beef tomatoes, red onion and garlic combined with fragrant fresh basil creates a truly delicious taste.'

4 **beef tomatoes** (the big ones!)
1 **vegetable stock cube**
1 tablespoon of **vegetable oil**
2 cloves of **garlic**, peeled and thinly chopped
1 small **red onion**, peeled and finely chopped
Freshly ground **black pepper**
Handful of fresh **basil**, chopped

1. Place the tomatoes in a large bowl.
2. Boil a kettle of water, pour over the tomatoes and leave for about 5 minutes.
3. Prepare the stock by dissolving the stock cube in ½ pint (285ml) of boiling water.
4. Carefully remove the tomatoes from the water, peel off the skins and chop the flesh into chunks.
5. In a large saucepan heat the oil and add the garlic, onion and tomatoes.
6. Gently sweat the vegetables over a medium heat for 10 minutes with the lid on.
7. Add the stock, seasoning and basil, bring to the boil and simmer for a further 15 minutes.
8. Remove from the heat and, using a blender (hand or jug), blend the soup briefly so that it retains a good texture.
9. Pour into a bowl and enjoy.

Why is this soup-a good for me? Tomatoes offer a range of amazing health benefits. Based on the volume of consumption per person, tomato is the top source of vitamins A and C in the Western diet. Unlike most foods, tomatoes are said to be more beneficial to health when cooked or processed. This is apparently because heat helps to break down the cell wall and release more of the phytochemical lycopene. Basil has antibacterial properties and contains flavonoids that help protect the cell structure.

Hunky Chunky Vegetable Soup

'A scrumptious vegetable soup containing hunky, chunky vegetables that simply melt in the mouth.'

1 **parsnip**
1 **carrot**
1 **sweet potato**
1 **leek**
1 **courgette**
1 **vegetable stock cube**
1 tablespoon of **vegetable oil**
Crushed **black pepper**

1. 'Top and tail' the parsnip, carrot, sweet potato, leek and courgette, peel and chop into small chunks.
2. Prepare the stock by dissolving the stock cube in 1 pint (570ml) of boiling water.
3. In a large saucepan heat the oil and add all the vegetables.
4. Gently sweat the vegetables over a medium heat for 15 minutes then add the stock and seasoning, bring to the boil and simmer for 10 minutes.
5. Remove from the heat and divide the soup roughly in half.
6. Blend one half of the soup (using a hand or jug blender), then combine the smooth soup with the chunky soup to create something smooth and creamy that you can really get your teeth into.

Why is this soup-a good for me? Carrots are a terrific source of anti-cancer betacarotene. Parsnips are particularly rich in vitamin C, potassium and calcium. Sweet potatoes have been found to help stabilize blood sugar levels and are also an excellent source of many antioxidants. Leeks could have the ability to reduce 'bad' LDL cholesterol levels and raise levels of 'good' HDL cholesterol.

Sweet Potato, Coconut and Chilli Soup

'Sweet potato and sublime coconut milk, subtly enriched with the rich spice of chilli.'

2 medium **sweet potatoes**
1 small **red chilli**, seeds removed
2 **spring onion** stalks
1 tablespoon of **vegetable oil**
1 can of half-fat **coconut milk**

1. Peel the sweet potatoes and chop into small chunks.
2. Chop the chilli and spring onion stalks into thin slices.
3. In a large saucepan heat the oil and add the sweet potatoes, chilli and onion.
4. Gently sweat the vegetables over a medium heat for 15 minutes then add the coconut milk and simmer for 10 minutes.
5. Remove from the heat and, using a blender (hand or jug), blend the soup until smooth.
6. Pour into a bowl and enjoy.

Why is this good for me? These two vegetables combined are excellent for helping to stabilize blood sugar levels. Onions are rich in chromium, a trace mineral that helps cells respond appropriately to insulin. Clinical studies of diabetics have shown that chromium can decrease fasting blood glucose levels, improve glucose tolerance, lower insulin levels, and decrease total cholesterol. Sweet potatoes are a good source of betacarotene and vitamin C. These powerful antioxidants work in the body to eliminate free radicals and therefore help prevent disease.

Pear and Parsnip Soup

'Firm pears and parsnips are the perfect partnership for this divine flavour sensation.'

2 **parsnips**
2 firm **pears**
1 **vegetable stock cube**
1 tablespoon of **vegetable oil**
1 small **red onion**, finely chopped
Crushed **black pepper**

1. 'Top and tail' the parsnips, then peel and chop into small chunks, including the core.
2. Peel the pears and cut the flesh into small chunks, discarding the core.
3. Prepare the stock by dissolving the stock cube in 1½ pints (850ml) of boiling water.
4. In a large saucepan heat the oil and add the onion and parsnips.
5. Gently sweat the vegetables over a medium heat for 15 minutes and then add the pear, stock and seasoning, bring to the boil and simmer for 15 minutes.
6. Remove from the heat and, using a blender (hand or jug), blend the soup until smooth.
7. Pour into a bowl and enjoy.

Why is this soup-a good for me? Parsnips are rich in potassium, calcium and vitamin C so are great for helping nerve function. Onions are a good source of chromium, a trace mineral that helps cells respond appropriately to insulin and therefore helps to stabilize blood sugar levels. Pears are a great source of dietary fibre as they contain the soluble fibre pectin which helps the body to eliminate toxins.

Soup-a-Juice

'This soup cleverly uses the pulp from the "Soup-a-Juice" (page 176), so it really is a "souperb" way of utilizing every little bit of goodness and fibre from the vegetables.'

1 **carrot**
1 **parsnip**
Pulp from **'Soup-a-Juice'** (page 176)
1 **stock cube**
1 tablespoon of **vegetable oil**
1 small **onion**, peeled and finely chopped
Crushed **black pepper**

1. 'Top and tail' the carrot and parsnip, then peel and chop into small chunks.
2. Prepare the stock by placing the pulp and a stock cube in a pan, adding 1 pint (570ml) of boiling water. Bring to the boil then simmer for 10 minutes.
3. Sieve the stock and throw away the residue pulp.
4. In a large saucepan heat the oil and add the carrot, parsnip and onion.
5. Gently sweat the vegetables over a medium heat for 15 minutes then add the stock and seasoning, bring to the boil and simmer for 10 minutes.
6. Remove from the heat and, using a blender (hand or jug), blend the soup until smooth.
7. Pour into a bowl and enjoy.

Why is this soup-a good for me? Carrots are one of the richest sources of vitamin A and betacarotene. They also contain vitamins B, C and K as well as a host of minerals such as calcium, potassium, magnesium, iron, phosphorous and sulphur. The calcium in carrots is more beneficial than calcium in milk or from supplements as the human body can absorb almost all of it. The nutrients in carrots help the efficient function of the immune, hormonal and nervous systems.

Onions contain vitamins B and C, the antioxidant quercetin, flavonoids and several other micronutrients which can help reduce blood clotting and raise healthy cholesterol.

Sweet Cherry Tomato and Roasted Pepper Soup

'Sweet cherry tomatoes and roasted peppers merge to create a souper-scrumptious flavour explosion. This soup is so delicious it's even made it into our Juice 'n' Smoothie Bars.'

1 **red pepper**
1 **yellow pepper**
1 small **red onion**
2 cloves of **garlic**, peeled
12 **cherry tomatoes**, stalks removed
1 tablespoon of **vegetable oil**
1 **vegetable stock cube**
Crushed **black pepper**

1. Preheat the oven to 180°C/350°F/Gas Mark 4.
2. Remove the stalks and seeds from the peppers and chop into small chunks.
3. Peel the onion and chop into chunks.
4. Place the peppers, onion, garlic and tomatoes on a large baking tray, drizzle with the oil and roast in the oven for 15 minutes.
5. Prepare the stock by dissolving the stock cube in 1 pint (570ml) of boiling water.
6. Remove the vegetables from the oven and empty into a large saucepan, add the stock and seasoning, bring to the boil and simmer for 10 minutes.
7. Remove from the heat and, using a blender (hand or jug), blend the soup until smooth.
8. Pour into a bowl and enjoy.

Why is this soup-a good for me? Peppers are high in vitamins C and B6 and bioflavonoids. They also contain capsaicin, a natural painkiller considered to be useful for arthritic pain. Red peppers contain lutein and zeaxanthin, which are useful for certain eye conditions. There is vitamin C in tomatoes as well as lycopene, a phytochemical with powerful anti-cancer properties. Once tomatoes have been heated, lycopene is more readily available to the body than in raw tomatoes.

Marvellous Magic Mushroom Soup

'The intense flavours of mushroom and garlic melted together and enveloped by smooth low-fat crème fraîche.'

250g **mushrooms**
2 cloves of **garlic**
1 small **red onion**
1 **vegetable stock cube**
1 tablespoon **vegetable oil**
Freshly ground **black pepper**
100g reduced-fat **crème fraîche**

1. Wash the mushrooms and chop into small chunks.
2. Peel the garlic and onion and chop into small pieces.
3. Prepare the stock by dissolving the stock cube in 1 pint (570ml) of boiling water.
4. In a large saucepan heat the oil and add the garlic, onion and mushrooms.
5. Gently sweat the vegetables over a medium heat for 10 minutes then add the stock and seasoning, bring to the boil and simmer for a further 10 minutes.
6. Remove from the heat, add the crème fraîche and, using a blender (hand or jug), blend the soup until smooth.
7. Pour into a bowl and enjoy.

Why is this soup-a good for me? This is so filling you won't have 'mushroom' for anything else! Like all vegetables, mushrooms are magic (sorry to disappoint if you actually thought this recipe contained real 'magic' mushrooms as in the type that make you feel like you're flying with Lord Lucan – for that you need to go to infamous Amsterdam).

Mushrooms are one of the few vegetables that should **NEVER** be juiced, so this recipe is great for exposing you to the many health benefits the humble mushroom has to offer. Mushrooms contain several key nutrients including selenium, copper, potassium, folate and niacin. Selenium is needed to help the antioxidant system function properly, and this is vital to help reduce the damaging effect of free radicals in the body. The mineral potassium helps the body maintain normal heart rhythm, fluid balance, and muscle and nerve function.

Spinach, Watercress, Rocket and Sweet Potato Soup

'Deep energetic spinach, watercress and rocket infused with the mellow flavours of dreamy sweet potato.'

1 small **red onion**
1 medium **sweet potato**
1 tablespoon **vegetable oil**
1 **vegetable stock cube**
Freshly ground **black pepper**
1 bag (140g) of **watercress**, **spinach** and **rocket**

1. Peel and chop the red onion and sweet potato into small pieces.
2. In a large saucepan heat the oil and add the onion and potato.
3. Gently sweat the vegetables over a medium heat with the lid on for 10 minutes.
4. Prepare the stock by dissolving the stock cube in 1 pint (570ml) of boiling water.
5. Add the stock, seasoning, spinach, watercress and rocket to the pan, bring to the boil and simmer for 5 minutes.
6. Remove from the heat and, using a blender (hand or jug), blend the soup until smooth.
7. Pour into a bowl and enjoy.

Why is this soup-a good for me? Spinach, watercress and rocket are all deep-green salad leaves and, as such, have many health benefits. They are packed with chlorophyll, the part of the plant that quite literally traps sunlight energy and releases it into your body's cells. Spinach contains many nutrients, the most famous being iron. Unfortunately, spinach is not the best source of iron for the body as it also contains substances that inhibit iron absorption. More importantly, spinach contains betacarotene and lutein, which is particularly important for the eyesight and for helping prevent cancer. Watercress is a brilliant source of vitamin C and magnesium as well as a good source of vitamins A, B1, B6 and E, betacarotene, iron, calcium and zinc.

17

Super-slimming Salads

All the salads contained in this section are incredibly simple to make yet delicious to devour. I adore nothing more than a big fresh salad packed with interesting and varied ingredients. If you think a salad consists of the abysmal effort that all too often gets served when dining out, prepare to be amazed!

Salads can be unbelievably dull, unappealing, tasteless, dry and unfulfilling. However, they can and *should be* exciting, tempting, bursting with delicious taste combinations and complemented with just the right dressing. Salads don't need to be complicated, and all too often the best ones are just the subtle combination of two or three ingredients. Again, I have added some nutritional info about each one so you have even more reason to tuck in.

Green Pesto Power Salad

'Avocado, cucumber and spring onion served on a bed of baby leaf spinach, rocket and watercress and drizzled with a pesto dressing.'

1 bag (140g) of **watercress**, **spinach** and **rocket** salad
1 large ripe **avocado**
¼ **cucumber**
2 **spring onion** stalks
100g **pesto**
2 tablespoons of extra virgin **olive oil**

1. Wash the salad leaves and place in a bowl.
2. Remove the flesh of the avocado, cut into generous slices and add to the salad.
3. Thinly slice the cucumber and spring onion stalks and add to the salad.
4. Empty the pesto into a small bowl, add the olive oil and mix well to create a dressing.
5. Pour the pesto dressing over the salad and serve.

Why is this SO good for me? Contrary to some misinformed beliefs, avocados are not a 'diet devil' food; they are in fact amazingly good for you. They are a complete food and contain an array of vitamins and minerals as well as essential fatty acids. Avocados contain 'good' fats that actually help regulate the appetite and prevent overeating, which means they satisfy the body and mind! Watercress, spinach and rocket are superb on the health front as the dark colours and distinctive flavours mean they are packed with phytonutrients (the disease-fighting nutrients). This is just a wonderful salad on every level, including – very importantly – the taste front!

Mozzarella, Beef Tomato and Basil Salad

'Simple soft buffalo mozzarella layered between juicy beef tomatoes and fresh basil, drizzled with extra virgin olive oil and balsamic vinegar.'

2 **beef tomatoes**
Small handful of fresh **basil**
150g fresh **buffalo mozzarella**
Extra virgin **olive oil**
Balsamic **vinegar**
Crushed **black pepper**

1. Wash the tomatoes and basil.
2. Cut the tomatoes and mozzarella into generous slices.
3. Layer the tomato, mozzarella and basil on a flat serving dish or plate.
4. Drizzle with olive oil and balsamic vinegar and sprinkle with freshly ground pepper.

Why is this SO good for me? This mouthwatering combination is an excellent source of vitamins A, B and C, calcium, potassium, phosphorus, antioxidants and betacarotene. Studies have shown that tomatoes provide powerful protection against many types of cancer due to the antioxidants they contain. They also contain a significant amount of dietary fibre.

This scrummy salad provides the body with a wonderful supply of amino acids (the building blocks of protein), which are essential for providing the body with structural integrity, transporting and storing nutrients, controlling growth and helping the immune system.

To make this vegan/vegetarian ... Simply leave out the cheese or replace with an alternative.

Baby Leaf Spinach, Mango, Blue Cheese and Toasted Pine Nut Salad

'Sweet baby leaf spinach accompanied by moist strips of mango and crumbled blue cheese, sprinkled with warm toasted pine nuts and dressed with rich balsamic vinegar.'

1 small bag (100g) of washed baby leaf **spinach**
½ ripe **mango**
150g **blue cheese**
50g **pine nuts**
Balsamic **vinegar**

1. Empty the bag of spinach into a bowl.
2. Peel the mango and cut into thin strips.
3. Cut the blue cheese into chunks.
4. Gently warm the pine nuts in a small pan.
5. Add the mango, blue cheese and pine nuts to the spinach.
6. Drizzle with balsamic vinegar and enjoy!

Why is this SO good for me? Mangos are an excellent source of vitamins A and C, as well as a good source of potassium and betacarotene. High in fibre but low in calories, they provide an additional sweet taste to this salad as well as a true nutritional boost. Pine nuts are a great source of carbohydrate and protein as well as calcium, phosphorus, iron and vitamins A, B1, B2 and B3. Spinach is a superb vegetable, rich in vitamins and minerals, particularly folate, vitamin K, magnesium and manganese.

This salad is high in vitamin A, which is particularly important for good vision, especially night vision.

To make this vegan/vegetarian ... Simply leave out the blue cheese or replace with an alternative.

Gorgeous Greek Salad

'Plump pitted olives and fresh crumbled feta combined with crisp cucumbers, peppers, onions and delicate baby tomatoes, tossed together with virgin olive oil and balsamic vinegar.'

150g **goats' cheese**
½ **red onion**
½ **red pepper**
½ **yellow pepper**
¼ **cucumber**
Large handful of plump pitted **olives**
Handful of baby **tomatoes**
Virgin **olive oil**
Balsamic **vinegar**
Freshly ground **black pepper**

1. Cut the goats' cheese, onion, peppers and cucumber into generous chunks and place in a salad bowl.
2. Add the olives and tomatoes and mix thoroughly.
3. Pour a generous glug of olive oil and balsamic vinegar over the salad.
4. Season with freshly ground black pepper.

Why is this SO good for me? Olives can count towards one of your five daily servings of fruit and vegetables, providing you eat about 10 olives. However, it is important to eat olives in small quantities because they are generally high in salt. Yellow and red peppers are full of essential nutrients, especially vitamin C. Interestingly, by weight, red peppers contain twice as much vitamin C as citrus fruit. Tomatoes are also high in vitamins C and A, as well as containing lycopene which can help prevent the development of cancer cells by neutralizing harmful free radicals.

In essence, all these raw vegetables contain a multitude of colours and thus phytonutrients, vitamins and minerals. As well as all its health benefits, this is a salad you can genuinely get your teeth into.

To make this vegan/vegetarian ... Simply leave out the blue cheese or replace with an alternative.

Warm Organic Chicken and Avocado Salad

'Warm organic chicken and ripe avocado served on a bed of wild rocket with shavings of Parmesan, sprinkled with fresh lemon juice and olive oil.'

2 skinless **chicken** breasts (preferably free range and organic)
1 bag (65g) of **wild rocket**
1 large ripe **avocado**
50g fresh **Parmesan**
1 **lemon**
Virgin **olive oil**

1. Grill the chicken for 20 minutes until cooked.
2. Meanwhile, wash the rocket and place in a salad bowl.
3. Remove the avocado flesh, chop into generous chunks and add to the rocket.
4. Remove the chicken from the grill, cut into generous chunks and add to the salad.
5. Using a peeler or sharp knife, shave thin slices of Parmesan over the salad.
6. Cut the lemon in half and squeeze the juice over the salad, along with a good drizzle of olive oil.

Why is this SO good for me? Wild rocket is a rich source of folate, calcium and iron as well as vitamins A and C. The phytochemicals that give rocket its bright green colour and distinctive flavour also help the body fight against disease. Avocados are a complete food and contain a multitude of nutritious benefits including essential fatty acids (EFAs), the 'good' fats! They are also an excellent source of carbohydrate, protein and dietary fibre. Interestingly, they contain about 60 per cent more potassium than bananas.

To make this vegan/vegetarian … Simply leave out the chicken or replace with an alternative.

Hot Honey Salmon Salad

'Delicate salmon drizzled with manuka honey and served on a bed of watercress, rocket, baby leaf spinach and cucumber.'

2 fresh **salmon** fillets
2 teaspoons of **manuka honey** (or other good-quality honey)
1 bag (140g) of **watercress**, **spinach** and **rocket** salad
½ **cucumber**
1 **lemon**
2 tablespoons of **balsamic vinegar**
2 tablespoons of virgin **olive oil**
Black **pepper**

1. Place the salmon (skin side up) on a piece of aluminium foil and cover each fillet with honey.
2. Grill the salmon for 10–15 minutes (do not turn over).
3. Meanwhile, wash the salad leaves and place in a bowl.
4. Thinly chop the cucumber and add to the salad.
5. Make up the dressing by combining the juice from the lemon with the balsamic vinegar, olive oil and pepper.
6. Drizzle the dressing over the salad and toss well.
7. Divide the salad onto 2 plates, remove the salmon from the grill and place directly on the prepared salads.

Why is this SO good for me? Salmon is an amazing source of high-quality protein as it contains all the essential amino acids, the building bricks for protein. Salmon also contains vitamins A, D, B6 and B2, as well as niacin, riboflavin, calcium, iron, zinc, magnesium and phosphorus. Above all, salmon is an excellent source of omega 3, an essential fatty acid (EFA) often missing from people's diets. The body cannot manufacture EFAs yet they are crucial for so many intrinsic processes, from regulating inflammation to supporting correct DNA function.

To make this vegan/vegetarian ... Simply leave out the salmon or replace with an alternative.

Winter Warmer Salad

'Oven-roasted butternut squash, peppers, red onion, courgette and baby tomatoes thrown on a bed of salad leaves dressed with avocado oil.'

2 tablespoons of **vegetable oil**
¼ butternut **squash**, peeled
½ **red pepper**
½ **yellow pepper**
1 small **red onion**, peeled
½ **courgette**
1 bag (100g) of mixed **salad leaves**
Avocado olive oil (or any oil of choice)
8 baby **tomatoes**
Black **pepper**

1. Preheat the oven to 180°C/350°F/Gas Mark 4.
2. Drizzle the oil onto a baking tray and warm in the oven for 10 minutes.
3. Roughly chop the butternut squash, peppers, onion and courgette into small chunks (about 1cm cubes), place on the baking tray and return to the oven for 25 minutes.
4. Wash the salad leaves, place in a bowl and drizzle with the avocado oil.
5. Remove the vegetables from the oven when ready, add the tomatoes, season with black pepper and return to the oven for a further 5 minutes.
6. When the vegetables are roasted remove from the oven and 'throw' over the prepared salad.

Why is this SO good for me? Squash is an excellent source of vitamin A (in the form of betacarotene), and a very good source of vitamin C, potassium, dietary fibre and manganese. In addition, squash is a good source of folate, omega 3 fatty acids, vitamins B1 and B6, copper and niacin. Peppers and tomatoes are full of essential nutrients, especially vitamins A and C. Vitamin A is needed for good vision, bone growth, reproduction and cell division. It also helps to regulate the immune system and promote a healthy surface lining for organs such as the eye and the respiratory, urinary and intestinal tracts.

Avocado, Alfalfa and Sun-blushed Tomato Salad

'Rich creamy avocado, accompanied by the delicate flavours of alfalfa sprouts and soft mellow sun-blushed tomatoes.'

1 bag (100g) of mixed **salad leaves**
50g **alfalfa sprouts**
100g sun-blushed **tomatoes** (you can use sun-dried if you prefer)
1 large ripe **avocado**
Juice of ½ **lemon**
2 tablespoons of virgin **olive oil**
2 tablespoons of **balsamic vinegar**

1. Wash the salad leaves and place in a bowl.
2. Add the alfalfa sprouts and sun-blushed tomatoes to the salad.
3. Remove the avocado flesh, chop into pieces and add to the salad.
4. Make up the dressing by combining the lemon juice, olive oil and balsamic vinegar.
5. Pour the dressing over the salad.

Why is this SO good for me? One of the most nutritionally concentrated sprouts, alfalfa sprouts contain high levels of protein, calcium, carotene, iron, magnesium, chlorophyll and potassium. They also have a high concentration of phytochemicals which can protect the body against diseases such as cancer, osteoporosis and cardiovascular diseases.

Avocados contain one of the highest levels of dietary fibre of any fruit and, interestingly, about 60 per cent more potassium than bananas.

Mixed Seed and Crunchy Vegetable Salad

'An array of crunchy vegetables, salad leaves and seeds, offering a multitude of textures and flavours to awaken the taste buds.'

1 bag of mixed **salad leaves**
½ small **red onion**, peeled
¼ **cucumber**
¼ **red pepper**
¼ **yellow pepper**
8 baby **tomatoes**
1 **carrot**
¼ small **red cabbage**
Extra virgin **olive oil**
Balsamic **vinegar**
1 small bag (100g) of **mixed seeds**

1. Wash the salad leaves and place in a bowl.
2. Thinly slice the onion, cucumber and peppers and add to the salad.
3. Chop the tomatoes in half and add to the salad.
4. Coarsely grate the carrot and cabbage directly into the salad.
5. Pour a generous glug of olive oil and balsamic vinegar over the salad.
6. Sprinkle the contents of the mixed seeds over the salad and enjoy.

Why is this SO good for me? Mixed seeds are a very good source of minerals such as phosphorous, magnesium, manganese, zinc, iron and copper. In addition, they are a good source of protein and vitamin K, carbohydrates, soluble and insoluble fibre, sodium, fatty acids, amino acids and more. Carrots are an excellent source of antioxidant compounds, and the richest vegetable source of the pro-vitamin A carotenes. The antioxidant compounds in carrots help protect against cardiovascular disease and cancer and also promote good vision, especially night vision. All the other vegetables are also rich in a multitude of vitamins, minerals, phytonutrients, enzymes and, of course, that intangible 'X-factor'.

Monkfish and Wild Rocket Salad

'Lightly grilled monkfish served with a wild rocket salad and drizzled with a honey and mustard dressing.'

1 bag (65g) of washed **wild rocket**
1 tablespoon of **honey** (manuka active honey is best)
1 teaspoon of **coarse-grain mustard**
2 tablespoons of extra virgin **olive oil**
200g fresh **monkfish**

1. Put the rocket into a bowl.
2. Mix together the honey, mustard and olive oil in a small bowl to make the dressing.
3. Cut the monkfish into chunks (about 10cm) and place on aluminium foil. Gently grill for 6–8 minutes.
4. Once cooked, add the monkfish to the rocket and drizzle the whole salad with the dressing.

Why is this SO good for me? Monkfish is an excellent low-fat, low-cholesterol source of protein. It is also high in selenium, niacin and vitamins B6 and B12. Manuka honey is indigenous to New Zealand, where it is made in the unpolluted forests. Active manuka is said to support the body's immune system in fighting a wide range of bacterial and fungal infections. Wild rocket is a rich source of iron as well as vitamins A and C, folate and calcium. It is also packed with phytochemicals which help the body fight disease.

To make this vegan/vegetarian ... Simply leave out the monkfish or replace with an alternative.

Something a Little Extra ...

Warm Stuffed Pittas

I have added this simply because it's a wonderful idea for lunch or dinner after the launch part of *Juice Yourself Slim*.

The best types are wholemeal pittas. There are several brands to choose from; my personal favourite are Marks and Spencer's own variety but any brand will do. This snack couldn't be easier – simply pop the pitta in the toaster and allow to warm through; once it's lightly toasted, cut along the long edge and stuff with any of the following, or a combination of your own.

Rocket, Sun-blushed Tomatoes, Olives and Feta Cheese

Simply stuff the pitta with the rocket, sun-blushed tomatoes, pitted olives and feta cheese (if you are vegan then omit the cheese).

Halloumi, Baby Leaf Spinach and Pesto

Slice the halloumi cheese and gently grill until browned. Use the pesto to 'butter' the pitta and then fill with the grilled halloumi and baby leaf spinach.

Avocado, Spinach, Cucumber and Spring Onion

Use the avocado to 'butter' the warm pitta and then stuff with sliced cucumber, spinach and spring onion.

Questions 'n' Answers

Can i have bread with my soup?

Ideally, for the launch programme, no. However, if you do choose to have some, make sure it's extremely good-quality, grainy bread. Rye bread is often better than wheat for many people. During the launch make sure you have only a couple of slices with the soup. It is all too easy to have half a loaf a night and wonder why you didn't drop the pounds required!

Can i microwave the soup?

It takes seconds to warm up soup in a pan so please keep soup out of the microwave where possible. If you have no choice then clearly, yes, warm it up in the microwave.

The recipes for the soups seem to make a lot. Do i need to eat all of it?

NO! The soup recipes are designed for two people. If you are not sharing your soup, keep half for the next day or simply make half the amount.

Do i have to keep to the juices, smoothies, soups and salads in this book?

Yes and no. Whilst on the seven-day launch programme it is important to stick with the recommended recipes as they have been carefully put together to ensure you have all your nutritional and dietary needs met. The juices, smoothies, soups and salads contain the right amount of good fats, protein, carbohydrates, fibre, vitamins and minerals. Once you are juicing yourself slim *for life* you are welcome to use any of the recipes in this book, or indeed make up a few of your own as long as they adhere to the same principles, and you don't start making up peanut butter smoothies or double cream leek and stilton soup!

What if i don't like a certain ingredient?

If there is a certain ingredient that you cannot stand, then feel free to leave it out or replace it with a similar ingredient. For example, substitute pears with apples or rocket with spinach. If you are not normally a fan of eating avocados I would urge you to try one of the recipes that contain blended avocados as they taste totally different in this form. Many people who would not normally eat an avocado seriously enjoy their mellow flavour once it's blended with gorgeous pineapple and other ingredients. If you really cannot stand avocado then omit it from the recipes but make sure you add a good source of omega 3, 6 and 9 oil to your soup or salad that day so you still get your essential fatty acids. I would recommend hemp oil. The other option is to use The Juice Master's Ultimate Juice Booster as it contains some good fats. The advantage of this is that it can be added directly to your juice, but I would always recommend blending it.

Can i swap juices, smoothies or soups during the launch if i don't like them?

Yes and no. Please feel free to swap any soup, and even have the same one every night if you wish. You will clearly have to adapt the shopping list. When it comes to smoothies and juices, I would strongly recommend that you keep to the programme. However, if you are going to swap, make sure you swap a fruit drink for another fruit drink, and a veggie drink for another veggie drink.

What else can i eat?

On the seven-day launch programme you should ideally eat nothing other than is outlined on the programme. However, after this initial launch you can eat whatever you desire as long as you adhere to the core principles (*page 137*). Clearly, if you have your two juices/smoothies per day and then eat nothing but junk for the rest of the day you won't be juicing yourself slim. My aim is that by the time you have read this book you will know what to feed yourself to fulfil genuine hungers and will not want to consume white refined sugars and fat on a daily basis.

Can i go out to eat during the launch?

Yes! Many people pick a week for the launch when they don't need to go out a great deal. However, you can still eat out and be successful. Most restaurants will have a good soup or a salad on the menu, and if you have had your juice/smoothie/juice during the day you will be fine.

⚉ What can i drink on the launch programme? Can i drink tea and coffee and what about alcohol?

Whenever you are thirsty, please feel free to drink as many herbal teas and as much mineral water as you like. As for tea, coffee and alcohol, for maximum results it is best not to have them during the seven-day launch. You will still lose a significant amount of weight even if you have the odd cup of coffee or glass of wine. However, to be free of all artificial stimulants during the launch will generate results far greater than just weight loss. It will also help to balance your body and enable you to distinguish between genuine hungers and false ones.

⚉ Can i do the programme without a juicer or blender?

Nope, you need both of these! The investment made is not just for the launch but for life.

⚉ What is the difference between a juicer and a blender?

A juicer or juice extractor extracts the liquid juice from the fibre of the fruit or vegetable, whereas a blender simply chops up the entire fruit and turns it into a yummy 'mush'. As a rule we tend to juice most vegetables and hard fruits and blend the soft fruits.

⚉ i own a blender. Do i still need to buy a smoothie maker?

No. Those sneaky boys and girls from a certain well-known company developed the 'smoothie maker' but this new machine is nothing more than a blender with a tap on it!

☘ it's annoying having to clean the juicer. is there any way around this?

Cleaning the machine can be a pain at times but these few tips should help:

- ☘ Place a bag in the pulp container (biodegradable ones are best) and then, after juicing, this can simply be thrown in the bin so the pulp container doesn't need cleaning.
- ☘ Always clean the juicer as soon as you have used it. This way the produce literally falls off the juicer with very little effort (except for the sieve, which just needs a little scrubbing with a small brush).
- ☘ You could make up all your juices for the day in one go and keep them in airtight flasks in the fridge (see page 161). This way you only need to clean the juicer once a day.
- ☘ You could pour some water through your juicer and turn it on for a few seconds after you have made a juice, and then it is okay to leave the juicer for a few hours before making the next juice. Having said that, this is a real lazy option and it is always better to clean your juicer immediately after using it.
- ☘ See juicemaster.com for tips on how to make a juice quickly!

☘ i'm on medication. it concerns me that you say all drugs are toxic and have adverse side-effects. Should i stop taking my medication and rely purely on juicing?

No, no and no again. In case you didn't hear me I said **NO, DO NOT STOP TAKING ANY MEDICATION WITHOUT SEEING YOUR GP FIRST.** I believe strongly in short-term medical intervention and I am far from being 'anti-doctor'. I am anti-**BIG MEDICINE** and their often underhand and manipulative ways. By incorporating juicing into your diet, one of the many positive side-effects is that you will be stocking up on Mother Nature's finest medicine, and over a period of weeks and months you should start to feel considerable changes to your health. The next time you visit your doctor for a checkup you should well find that certain conditions have improved and that your regular prescriptions may need to be significantly adjusted.

☺ Can i do the programme if i am pregnant?

During your first 12 weeks of pregnancy you are advised not to change anything much about your diet or lifestyle, so if this programme is a radical change for you then it's best not to start it as suffering detox symptoms on top of morning sickness is probably not a good idea. During your pregnancy you shouldn't be looking to lose weight, and most people embark on this programme after the baby is born. As always, please consult your GP.

☺ Can i continue with the launch programme for longer than seven days?

Yes and indeed yes again. Unlike the *7lbs in 7 Days* book where all you could consume for 7 days was juices and smoothies, this programme is different. The launch can be continued for as long as you like. I know many people who were so happy doing the launch that they now incorporate this into their daily lifestyle. Many people 'launch' themselves from Monday to Friday and then eat pretty much what they like over the weekend. Interestingly, even at weekends they often continue to have a juice or smoothie each day. These people are certainly not 'on a diet'. They have genuinely changed their diet and to this day, despite being slim, they are still living a *Juice Yourself Slim* lifestyle.

✌ Can i do the programme by using shop-bought 100-per-cent fruit and vegetable juices and smoothies?

No, I'm afraid not. Did you read the rest of this book! The juices and smoothies you make at home and those found in the chiller cabinet of your local supermarket are worlds apart on the nutrition front. The legal requirement of heat-treating and pasteurizing the bottled juice means that lots of the vitamins and minerals are destroyed, together with life-giving enzyme activity. You will still get some goodness from these drinks but you could and should not rely on them wholly. In case of an 'emergency' you could substitute one of the juices or smoothies on the programme with a bottled option; however, this really should be an exception and not the rule. The Innocent brand is one of the best out there – always worth paying a bit more!

✌ Can i get my juices and smoothies from a juice bar?

This really does depend on the type of juice bar you visit. If there is a Juice Master Juice 'n' Smoothie Bar near you then you can be guaranteed to find a range of fresh vegetables and fruits just waiting to be juiced. Genuine juice bars will offer fruit and vegetable juices and smoothies made using freshly extracted juice. This is really, really important as many use 'ready-made' juice that sits at the back of the bar somewhere in a cooler. This juice is almost always not freshly extracted and is often concentrated or pasteurized. Another thing to look for is smoothies that are laden with sugar-filled yoghurt. Often, juice bars will claim to make all their smoothies with 'fat-free' or '98 per cent fat-free' yoghurt, which looks good on the surface. However, if you dig a little deeper you will discover that they are often made with yoghurt which can contain up to 40 per cent sugar. Just keep vigilant as not all juices and smoothies are as innocent as they first appear. *(See page 285 for a list of good juice bars.)*

🏋 What if i really cannot make or buy a fresh juice/smoothie?

It's always worth remembering that we all own a personal blender and juice extractor in the form of our teeth and digestive system. At times when you simply cannot use a juicer or find a genuine juice bar then I would suggest buying some locally grown or organic fruit and eating it. When on the move I usually grab a bunch of grapes or a couple of juicy oranges to keep me nourished. The only time I would say to steer away from this option is if you are on a long journey and the only fruit you can get your hands on is the shrivelled-up or plastic-looking variety found in garages and service stations. Ideally, prepare for a long journey by making up a juice/smoothie in advance (*see page 161*). In these circumstances, as mentioned above, I would opt for buying a good quality *innocent*-looking smoothie. To top up your nutritional bank account at times when you cannot juice, I recommend that you mix some Juice Master's Ultimate Superfood or Ultimate Boost Juice with water (*see page 163*). This is vital to replenish the vitamins, minerals and enzymes that you will be missing out on.

🏋 i'm suffering from headaches. is this normal?

Believe it or not, this is a good sign as it means you are withdrawing from drugs or drug-like substances. Like any drug, when you stop taking things such as caffeine, alcohol, nicotine and sugars you will suffer a degree of withdrawal which will manifest itself as headaches or even anxiety. It is worth mentioning here that the reason you are feeling such symptoms is not because you are low on the particular substance/s but because you took them in the first place. This is a natural part of the healing process and should only last for a few days, after which time you will feel like a brand new you.

🜚 i'm suffering from tiredness and low energy levels. is this normal?

Again, this is a good sign as it means your body is eliminating toxins. Depending on how 'toxic' you are, you may well find you start experiencing headaches or problem skin. Because you aren't stuffing the body with artificial stimulants you won't be subject to instant caffeine and sugar highs. These unnatural highs are all too often followed by massive lows, which then create more of a false need for the same artificial substance to make you feel 'normal' again. When you stop falsely stimulating the body it takes a little time for it to find its natural equilibrium and for you to tap into your natural energy source. Again, this is a very natural part of the healing process and in no time at all you will feel a wonderful natural high without relying on artificial substances.

🜚 i'm feeling sick and i've got stomach cramps. is this normal?

No, this is not normal. Sickness can occur when you first go on a juice plan but this shouldn't last longer than a day. One of the reasons might be that you are drinking your juices and smoothies too quickly. Always 'chew' your drinks as the digestive enzymes in your mouth are stronger than those in your stomach. Look at what is going into your juices and smoothies and accept that you wouldn't simply swallow these foods down in one mouthful. Be sensible and savour your juices and smoothies. If you do this and are still feeling nauseous after day one then come off the plan **IMMEDIATELY** and see your GP as soon as possible.

✋ My poo is sometimes red. Should i worry?

Your poo may well turn red if you are consuming juices that contain a lot of raw beetroot, and clearly this is nothing to be concerned about. The other reason why your poo might be red is because you have haemorrhoids; again, this is not too serious and is usually caused by a burst blood vessel as a result of 'straining' too hard. This usually repairs itself within a couple of days but if the problem persists go and see you GP to get it checked out.

✋ Will i get all of my five-a-day in just one juice or smoothie?

Hmm, this is a tricky one. If you take five or more fruits and vegetables that will be used to make a smoothie and consume them all then you have officially met the government's recommended five-a-day policy. However, if you take these exact same ingredients and put them into a blender with some freshly extracted apple or pineapple juice then for some reason they magically metamorphose into just one portion. Although on the surface this very limited categorization system may make it seem that the government has a vendetta against juices and smoothies, the reality is that this blanket label is applied to all juices and smoothies – both the freshly made variety and those bought in bottles. So technically, if you make the smoothie yourself you 'know' how many portions you are getting. However, if you buy one it really can count as only one portion.

✋ Will the programme still work for me even if i don't exercise?

Yes, you will still get great results even if you do not exercise. However, you will get *amazing* results if you exercise too. Exercise not only gets your body in great shape but it also releases endorphins which instantly make you feel good. If you do not exercise then you will not lose as much weight and you will also not feel as good as if you get your body moving and heart pumping twice a day.

♉ How much weight should i expect to lose during the launch?

On average you should expect to lose around 7lbs providing you follow the programme to the letter. If you choose not to stick to the programme 100 per cent, or you do not exercise twice a day, then you may well lose less. People with more weight to lose may in fact lose more than 7lbs, and if you do then this is nothing to be concerned about.

♉ i did the programme but i didn't lose much/any weight.

The best time to weigh yourself is the night before you start the programme and then again on the morning of Day 8. On average, you should expect to lose around 7lbs. However, sometimes there is a time lag and this weight loss may appear one, two or three days after you have finished the launch. If you do not lose any more weight in this time then it's probably because you don't need to and your body has found its natural weight. If you feel that you truly are overweight and have followed the plan to the letter then it might be that you are one of the very few people with a genuine thyroid problem and you should get yourself checked out by your GP.

That should be it, but no doubt by the time you read this many people will have written in with more questions, so for more questions 'n' answers go to juicemaster.com

Recommended Juice and Smoothie Bars

💪 Juice Master Juice 'n' Smoothie Bars

The reason I started my own chain of juice and smoothie bars was simply in response to what was out there. I was genuinely fed up with juice bars hoodwinking the public with the illusion of 'fresh' and 'healthy'. Many juice bars use sugar-loaded yoghurt and pasteurized juices for all their smoothies. I wanted to make sure that when you go into a juice bar the health has been taken care of for you. The Juice Master chain of juice bars is growing fast and a full list is found at juicemaster.com. If you want to get involved in the juice revolution yourself and are interested in opening your own juice bar, simply contact our team at **info@juicemaster.com**. We opened our first one in Leeds University and have since opened two in Waterford in Ireland. By the time you read this book there will be many more …

18 John Roberts Square, Waterford, Ireland

Ardkeen Quality Food Store, Ardkeen, Waterford, Ireland

Other Great Juice Bars

Not all juice bars out there are bad. In fact, there are some extremely good ones. Here are a few …

B Juicy, Truro in Cornwall. This is not a juice bar chain and is the only juice bar in Truro at the time of writing. It serves great juice and the person who runs it has a genuine passion for the subject.

The Big Banana, Bristol. A great juice bar owned by John LeFevre. Probably the best wheatgrass juice in the country … other than ours clearly!

St Nicholas Market, Unit 21 The Glass Arcade, St Nicholas's Market, Corn Street, Bristol BS1 1LG. The original juice bar, established in the summer of 2001. Open Monday to Friday 7.30am to 5pm and on Saturday from 8am to 5pm.

Juice Moose, Exeter and Plymouth

Want to be a Juice Master Natural Juice Therapist?

Due to the genuine health benefits of natural juice therapy and my passion to get this alternative treatment not so 'alternative', I am proud to present the first ever 'Juice Therapist' accreditation. This is a unique opportunity to become an official Juice Master Natural Juice Therapist.

My mission is to 'juice the world', and it's a difficult task to accomplish alone. This is why I am looking for genuine, compassionate and caring individuals to join me on this incredibly rewarding path. If this is something that genuinely juices you, please email us or see juicemaster.com for full details.

The course has been accepted by the CMA (Complementary Medicine Association) and accredited by an English university.

Index

Recipes are shown in **bold**

acai 166, 203
acrylamide 80–1
adverse drug reactions (ADRs) 13–14
Ahluwalia, Amrita 58
alfalfa sprouts 266–7
alkaline (pH) balance 179, 181, 189, 190
Alli weight-loss pill 16–17
Alzheimer's disease 53–4
amino acids 23, 171, 175, 205, 223, 255, 263, 269
Aniston, Jennifer 9, 99
antioxidants 21, 54, 55, 56, 61, 108, 166, 171, 179, 190, 191, 197, 199, 208, 213, 217, 224, 233, 239, 241, 245, 255, 269
Apple 'n' Pear Zesty Twist 178
apples 21, 54, 57, 59, 60, 173, 176–7, 178, 179, 180, 184–5, 188–9, 190, 191, 193, 194–5, 196–7, 198–9, 208, 210–11, 212, 213, 214, 216–17, 218–19, 220, 222–3, 224, 226–7, 228–9, 230
  and asthma 52–3
  nutritional depletion 81, 103–4, 166
arthritis 26, 31, 59, 79, 172, 185, 191, 207, 235

aspartame 25, 82
aspirin therapy 51
asthma 28, **44–5**, 52–3, 78, 185, 207
Atkins diet 13, 93–4
Avocado, Alfalfa and Sun-blushed Tomato Salad 266–7
avocados 201, 204–5, 206–7, 212, 214, 215, 218–19, 222–3, 225, 253, 260–1, 266–7, 272, 274

Baby Leaf Spinach, Mango, Blue Cheese and Toasted Pine Nut Salad 256–7
bananas 202–3, 209, 218–9, 220, 224, 226–7
basil 236–7, 254–5
Beckham, Victoria 30, 35
beetroot 173, 191, 212
  and hypertension 58–9
berries 60, 216–17, 221
  see also blueberries; cranberries; strawberries
Beta-Carrot Juice 173
betacarotene 57, 71, 166, 173, 179, 182, 186, 191, 208, 212, 223, 227, 233, 239, 241, 245, 251, 255, 257, 265
Bio-live Berries 221
bladder cancer 66
blame culture 112

blenders/smoothie makers 152, 276
Blood Builder 212
blue cheese 256–7
blueberries 60, 196–7, 202–3, 208, 228–9
Blueberry Power 208
BMI index 22
Body Balancer 181
boosters 73–4, 167–8, 205
breast cancer 61–2
broccoli 105, 174–5, 198–9, 204–5,
    234–5
bromelain 186, 187, 195
Burney, Peter 53
butternut squash 232–3, 264–5
**Butternut Squash and Carrot Soup
    232–3**

calcium 71, 72, 104, 179, 181, 189, 209,
    213, 214, 221, 223, 229, 230, 235,
    239, 243, 245, 251, 255, 257, 261,
    263, 267, 271
cancer 26, 79, 95, 102
    and carrots 48–9, 57–8, 173, 186
    and cooked food 80–1
    prevention 21, 89, 185, 190, 197, 224,
        227, 233, 247, 251, 255, 259, 267,
        269
    see also specific cancers
Cantaloupe Cooler 182
cantaloupe melon 182
Canter, Dr 15
capsaicin 191, 245
carbohydrates 23, 214, 217, 257, 261,
    269
Carroll, Kenneth 61
Carrot 'n' Pineapple Twist 186
carrots 173, 176–7, 183, 186, 212,
    232–3, 238–9, 244–5, 268–9
    and cancer 48–9, 57–8, 173, 186
celery 59, 60, 181, 188–9, 198–9, 214,
    222–3, 234–5
Changing Diets approach 115–16
Changing Rooms 114–15, 119, 147
cherries 59–60
chicken 260–1
chillies, red 240–1
chlorine 189, 230

chlorophyll 48, 49, 175, 199, 251, 267
cholesterol 17–18, 207
    and citrus juice 61
    and heart disease 69–70
    HDL 235, 239, 245
    LDL 26, 61, 70, 235, 239
    and phytosterols 229
    statins vs. juicing 31
chromium 241, 243
cinnamon 194–5
co-factors 58, 103, 165
coconut milk 240–1
colon cancer 185, 235
cooked food 80–1, 86
copper 187, 189, 233, 249, 265, 269
core principles 136–45
courgettes 174–5, 176–7, 188–9,
    210–11, 234–5, 238–9, 264–5
cranberries 54, 193, 220
Cranberry Banana Blend 220
crème fraîche 248–9
Crozier, Alan 54
**Cucumber, Apple 'n' Kiwi Cooler
    184–5**
Cucumber Shake 210–11
cucumbers 59, 60, 174–5, 181, 183,
    184–5, 188–9, 198–9, 210–11, 214,
    215, 218–19, 222–3, 225, 253,
    258–9, 262–3, 268–9, 272
Currie, Edwina 18

dairy intolerance 94
Dead Sea treatment 19
diabetes 26, 195, 241
'diet' mentality 1, 14, 91, 122–3, 144
dietary fibre 211, 223, 233, 243, 255,
    261, 265, 267, 269
'diets', blaming 112
digestive restriction 103
drinks 276
drug (junkie) foods 1–2, 4, 78, 81–3,
    99–100, 101, 123–6, 145–6
drug (pharmaceutical) industry 11–28,
    71–4, 229

eating out 275
eczema 79

egg 'health crisis' 18
ellagic acid 208, 221
emotional eating 139
endometriosis 41–2
endorphins 107, 108, 142, 164
energy bars 164
energy loss 132, 281
enzymes 103, 171, 175, 190, 207, 224, 269
erectile dysfunction 56
essential fatty acids (EFAs) 17, 166, 201, 205, 207, 214, 219, 223, 225, 229, 253, 261, 263, 269, 274
European Nutrition and Health Claims Regulations 69
'everlasting light bulbs' 87
exercise 43–4, 106–13, 142, 157, 282
  beneficial juices 60
  equipment 153–4

falcarinol 57, 173
fats *see* essential fatty acids; trans fats
fennel 215
Fennel Fuel 215
feta cheese 272
five-a-day 59, 282
flasks 153, 161
flavonoids 51, 53, 59, 60, 61–2, 237, 245, 247
Flora pro.activ 69–70
folate 179, 209, 211, 214, 233, 235, 249, 257, 261, 265, 271
folic acid 208, 211
Folts, John D 50–1
Food and Drug Administration (FDA) 21
'food freedom' mentality 1–2, 91, 123–6, 144
food industry 69–70, 81–3, 145–6
Food Standards Agency (FSA) 17, 73, 80, 82
Forest, Christopher 56
free radicals 21, 54, 108, 182, 185, 187, 190, 191, 212, 241, 249, 259
Fruity Bio-live Breakfast Smoothie 216–17
Fruity Rescue Remedy 192
Fruity Superfood Sensation 202–3

garlic 236–7, 246–7, 248–9
ginger 187, 188–9, 209
Ginger Orange Smoothie 209
global warming 76–7, 92
goats' cheese 258–9
goji berries 166, 202–3, 226–7
  call for ban 71
Goji Berry Bonanza 226–7
Gorgeous Greek Salad 258–9
gout 26, 59–60
Grace, Janey Lee 109
Grand Design approach 47, 115–16, 117–19
Grand Designs 115, 119, 128
grapefruit
  and breast cancer 61–2
  and osteoporosis 61
grapes (red/purple) 54, 190, 196–7
  vs. wine 50–2
Green Pesto Power Salad 253
Green Slimming Fuel 174–5
greenhouse gases 93
Guinness 52, 183
Guthrie, Najla 61–2

halloumi 272
Halvorsen, Richard 18
hand blenders 152
hay fever 33–4
headaches 33–4, 132, 280
health
  insurance 96–105
  and juicing 6–7, 11–12, 24–5, 47–9, 50–68, 77–9, 88, 92, 102–5
heart disease 13, 17–18, 26, 79, 95, 102, 185, 190, 227, 235
  and cholesterol 69–70
  grape juice vs. wine 50–2
  and pomegranate juice 56
Hensrud, Donald 16–17
high blood pressure
  see hypertension
Hippocrates 61
honey 224, 262–3, 270–1
Hot Honey Salmon Salad 262–3
hunger
  and emotions 139

and exercise 107
induced by big foods 81–3, 145–6
mental 133
and nutritional shortage 81, 91
and withdrawal 131–2
Hunky Chunky Vegetable Soup
  238–9
hyperactivity 25, 26
hypertension 13, 15, 26
  and beetroot 58–9
hypnosis 5–6

IBS 79, 215
inspirational fire 1–8, 27, 28–9, 31,
  46–7, 130, 142–3
internal environment 77–9, 89–92
iron 52, 71, 74, 173, 179, 183, 189, 191,
  213, 214, 221, 223, 227, 229, 230,
  235, 245, 251, 257, 261, 263, 267,
  269, 271

Jarvis, Dr 27
Jensen, Bernard 48, 77–8, 92
juice bars 162–3, 279, 285–6
  in hospitals 34, 45–6
juice extractors (juicers) 7, 30, 111,
  150–2, 276
  cleaning 277
Juice Master
  Berry Boost 153, 203, 221
  boosters and supplements 73–4, 153,
    167–8
  Clear Skin Boost 74, 153, 225
  Energy bars 164
  Juice 'n' Smoothie Bars 163, 279
  Natural Juice Therapists 67, 287
  Ultimate Detox Boost 153, 181
  Ultimate Juice Boost 153, 164, 205,
    207, 274, 280
  Ultimate Superfood 153, 164, 207,
    280
  Variety Pack 153, 167
juices
  boosters 165–8
  'juice league' 84–5
  nutritional balance 85–6
  recipes 171–99

shop-bought 83–4, 279
juicing
  and health 6–7, 11–12, 24–5, 47–9,
    50–68, 77–9, 88, 92, 102–5
  for life 114–19, 136–49
  on the move 160–4, 280
  reasons for 102–5
  scientific studies 50–62
  test programme 40, 62–7
  and weight loss 9–11, 26, 28, 30–47,
    89–91
  testimonials 24, 30–47, 90–1, 63–6,
    148–9
Jordan 9, 35, 37

kale 174–5
Kendrick, Malcolm 70
Kirschner, H E 48
kiwis 184–5

labelling 140–1
launch 129–30, 131–4
  essential equipment 150–3
  optional extras 153–4
  preparation 133–5
  questions and answers 273–83
  seven-day programme 157–9
  shopping list 155–6
leeks 57, 234–5, 238–9
lemons 21–2, 59, 173, 178, 183, 186,
  188–9, 191, 192, 202–3, 204–5,
  210–11, 212, 224, 260–1, 262–3,
  266–7
leptogenic society 75
life expectancy 118
limes 174–5, 179, 180, 192, 206–7, 215,
  225, 230
lutein 251
lycopene 237, 247, 259
lymph system 98, 106–7

magnesium 104, 179, 186, 189, 221,
  229, 230, 245, 251, 257, 263, 267,
  269
malic acid 180
manganese 179, 233, 235, 257, 265, 269
mangetout peas 198–9

Mango and Honey Zest 224
mangos 21, 213, 224, 265–7
manuka honey 208, 262–3, 270–1
marathon running 40, 110, 219
Marvellous Magic Mushroom Soup
   248–9
meat and dairy 93–5
medication 277–8
mental factors 1–2, 14, 27–8, 114,
   122–8
migraines 43–4, 70
minerals 23, 58, 92, 103, 171, 175, 177,
   179, 183, 191, 199, 205, 212, 217,
   223, 224, 253, 259, 269
mini-trampolines 109–10, 140
mint 230
Mixed Seed and Crunchy Vegetable
   Salad 268–9
MMR vaccine 18
monkfish 270–1
Monkfish and Wild Rocket Salad
   270–1
Moore, Michael 96, 97
Moss, Kate 30
mozzarella 254–5
Mozzarella, Beef Tomato and Basil
   Salad 254–5
MP3/MP4 players 141
muesli 216–17
muscle pain 59–60
mushrooms 248–9

NASA (Never Accept Stereotypical
   Assumptions) 120–2
Natural Skin Boost 225
NHS 75, 96–7
nitrate 58
nutritional depletion 81, 103–4, 165–6
nutritional investment 102–5

obesity and overweight 70, 86
  advantages 126–8
  blame culture 112
  'cure' 14, 16
  as 'disease' 20–2
  epidemic 26, 68
  fat pressure cycle 116–17

  and food addiction 14, 27
  'getting away with it' 101
  obesogenic society 74–5
older people 31, 34
olives 258–9, 272
omega 3 217, 233, 263, 265, 274
omega 6 217, 274
omega 9 217, 274
'one disease' hypothesis 77–8
onions 244–5
  red 232–3, 236–7, 242–3, 246–7, 248–9,
   250–1, 258–9, 264–5, 268–9, 242–3
oranges 21, 192, 202–3, 209
  and breast cancer 61–2
  and osteoporosis 61
Orchard Delight 190
Organic Avocado Crush 206–7
organic fruit snacks 160–1
'organic' labels 141
organic vs. 'normal' health care 105–6
osteoporosis 60–1, 107, 172, 235, 267
overeating 139–40

Pantuck, Allan 55
Parmesan 260–1
parsnips 173, 176–7, 238–9, 242–3,
   244–5
Pasteur, Louis 77
Pear, Pineapple and Ginger Juice 187
Pear and Parsnip Soup 242–3
pears 21, 178, 187, 190, 193, 242–3
pectin 178, 185, 187, 189, 193, 230, 243
Pepper Punch 191
peppers
  red 191, 246–7, 258–9, 264–5, 268–9
  yellow 188–9, 191, 246–7, 258–9,
   264–5, 268–9
personal health care 97–102
personality 127–8
pesto 253, 272
pharmaceuticals see drug industry
phen-phen 13
phosphorus 189, 221, 229, 230, 245,
   255, 257, 263, 269
phytonutrients 53, 191, 197, 199, 205,
   212, 214, 217, 223, 235, 253, 259,
   261, 267, 269, 271

phytoestrogens 217
pine nuts 256–7
Pineapple, Mint and Lime Shake 230
Pineapple 'n' Cinnamon Spice 194–5
pineapples 174–5, 179, 181, 183, 186, 187, 192, 193, 194–5, 198–9, 204–5, 206–7, 215, 220, 221, 225, 230
Pitt, Brad 22
polycystic ovarian syndrome (PCOS) 63–4
polyphenols 53, 54, 56, 104, 190, 197
pomegranates 60, 202–3
   and heart disease 56
   and prostate cancer 55–6
   recipe 202–3
Pondimin 13
poo, red 282
potassium 60, 177, 181, 186, 189, 211, 213, 219, 221, 223, 224, 230, 239, 243, 245, 249, 255, 257, 261, 265, 267
power greens 163–4
pregnancy 179, 211, 278
prostate cancer 55–6
protein 223, 229, 257, 261, 267, 269, 271
   animal 93–5
   digestion 186, 195, 207
psoriasis 19, 74, 97
Purple Power 196–7

quinine 193, 220

raw food 79–80, 81, 86–7
rebounding 108–10
red cabbage 57, 268–9
rocket 214, 250–1, 253, 260–1, 262–3, 270–1, 272
Rocket Fuel 214
Rooker, Jeff 72–3
Rubik's Cube 121–2
Ryan, Keith 142

salad leaves 264–5, 266–7, 268–9
salad recipes 251–71
salmon 262–3

Savoury Superfood Sensation 204–5
science 28, 67–8
scurvy 21, 192
seeds, mixed 268–9 *see also* sesame seeds; sunflower seeds
Seedy Summer Berry Crush 228–9
selenium 71, 104, 165, 249, 271
self-help 129–30
sesame seeds 228–9
7lbs in 7 Days Super Juice Diet 9, 11, 24, 47
shop-bought juices 83–4, 279
sickness 282
SiCKO 96
silica 189, 211
Sixth Sense Syndrome 3–4
skin conditions 19, 47, 74, 78
Slim 4 Life 1, 2–3
Slimline Tonic 180
Smith, Ian 57
smoking 3–4, 27, 70, 83, 99, 100–1, 131–2
smoothie recipes 200–30
snacks and snacking 140, 160–1
sodium 60, 181, 189, 224, 269
soup
   questions and answers 273
   recipes 231–51
Soup-a-Juice (juice) 176–7
Soup-a-Juice (soup) 244–5
'Souper' Green Stuff 234–5
Spies, Tom 89
spinach 21, 59, 174–5, 179, 181, 183, 198–9, 204–5, 210–11, 222–3, 234–5, 250–1, 253, 256–7, 262–3, 272
Spinach, Watercress, Rocket and Sweet Potato Soup 250–1
Spinach Stout 183
spirit 157–8
spirulina 73–4, 166, 167, 175, 222–3
Spirulina Smoothie 222–3
spring onions 240–1, 253, 272
sprouts (sprouted seeds) 204–5
Spurlock, Morgan 62–3
statins 31, 70
strawberries 213, 228–9

Strawberry and Mango Melt 213
sulphur 189, 230, 245
sunflower seeds 228–9
Sunny Delight 73
Super Juice Me! test programme 40,
  62–7
Super Sporty Fuel Smoothie 218–19
superfoods 166
supplements
  bans 71–3
  for juices 72–3, 165–8, 205
Sweet Cherry Tomato and Roasted
  Pepper Soup 246–7
Sweet 'n' Savoury 179
Sweet Potato, Coconut and Chilli
  Soup 240–1
sweet potatoes 238–9, 240–1, 250–1
Sweet Veggie Heaven 188–9

Taylor, E. 67
Taylor, Victoria 58–9
teenagers 35
testimonials 24, 30–47, 90–1, 148–9
Tomato and Basil Soup 236–7
tomatoes
  baby 258–9, 264–5, 268–9
  beef 236–7, 254–5
  cherry 246–7
  sun-blushed 266–7, 272
trans-fats 17–18, 152

Uncle Fred Syndrome 99–102
US health care 96

Very Tart Tonic, A 193
Vioxx 15
vitamins 23, 58, 92, 103, 171, 175, 177,
  179, 183, 191, 199, 205, 212, 217,
  223, 224, 233, 259, 269
  A 17, 179, 180, 182, 189, 209, 211,
    213, 214, 224, 230, 237, 235, 245,
    251, 253, 255, 257, 259, 261, 263,
    265, 271
  B 12, 180, 186, 189, 191, 208, 209,
    213, 221, 229, 230, 235, 245, 255
  B1 179, 251, 257, 265
  B2 (riboflavin) 71, 257, 263

  B3 (niacin) 233, 249, 257, 263, 265,
    271
  B6 72–3, 179, 233, 247, 251, 263, 265,
    271
  B12 271
  C 71–2, 179, 180, 182, 185, 186, 187,
    189, 191, 192, 203, 208, 209, 211,
    213, 214, 221, 224, 227, 230, 233,
    235, 237, 239, 241, 243, 245, 247,
    251, 255, 257, 259, 261, 265, 271
  D 17, 263
  E 17, 179, 186, 189, 221, 223, 229,
    251
  K 17, 179, 186, 235, 245, 257, 269
  supplement bans 71–3

wall planners 153
Warm Organic Chicken and Avocado
  Salad 260–1
Warm Stuffed Pittas 272
watercress 174–5, 179, 198–9, 250–1,
  253, 262–3
weight loss
  alternative remedies 14–15
  during launch 283
  and juicing 9–11, 26, 28, 30–47,
    89–91
  quick results 11, 36
  simple way 120–30
  testimonials 30–47, 90–1, 148–9
weight-loss drugs 12–28, 68
wheatgrass 30, 175
  powder 153, 175
wild animals 79, 86, 111
wine vs. grape juice 50–2
Winter Warmer Salad 264–5
World Health Organization 26, 46
World's Your Oyster, The 198–9

X factor 62, 79, 81, 86, 104, 171, 199,
  212, 269

yoghurt, bio-live 208, 213, 216–17, 221,
  226–7

zinc 71, 165, 179, 213, 225, 229, 251,
  263, 269

Juicy Info

For more information on the Juice Booster range, Juice Master books, CDs, DVDs, forthcoming seminars, juice-bar opportunities, plus anything else you need to know about our juicy world, please contact us at:

Juice Master Hotline: **08451 30 28 29**
(this is a local call charge from anywhere in the UK)
Website: **www.juicemaster.com**
E-mail: **info@juicemaster.com**

The Juice Master's Mind and Body Detox Retreats

Fancy an amazing experience? Why not spend a week in a beautiful European coastal destination, drinking only the finest-quality freshly extracted juices, doing yoga, meditation, meeting new people and attending seminars designed to change the way you think about what you feed yourself? These are only held a few times a year, so places go fast. For more info, see the website or speak to one of the juicy team. Use the juicy vouchers to get you started!

Happy juicing!

Buy 1 Get 1 Free at any Juice Master Juice Bar (at all participating outlets)	**£75 OFF** 1-Week Detox Retreat	**£75 OFF** 3-Day Juice/ Spa Detox

Note: The money off vouchers are not in conjunction with any other offer.

Printed by RR Donnelley at Glasgow, UK